# Rethinking Alzheimer's Care

*The authors challenge professionals across care settings to deepen our thinking about why and what we do with people with Alzheimer's disease and their families. This is a soulful look at the values and practice of dementia care. Fazio, Seman, and Stansell have made a significant contribution to the growing literature on person-centered care.*

Daniel Kuhn, M.S.W.
Education Director, Rush Alzheimer's Disease Center

*Thought-provoking, inspirational and upbeat approach to caring ABOUT people with Alzheimer's and their families across settings. Builds upon Kitwood's unfinished work with real-world examples that inspire us to look beyond labels for the person and the meaning. [An] important message about caring from seasoned authors who do care.*

Lisa P. Gwyther, M.S.W.
Director, Duke Family Support Program, Duke University Medical Center

*A visionary book from three leaders in the field of dementia care, chock full of ideas for rethinking our services for people with dementia.*

David Troxel, M.P.H.
Executive Director, Santa Barbara Alzheimer's Association, and co-author,
*The Best Friends Approach to Alzheimer's Care*

*In this new book, the reader will discover how the person with dementia can "step forward" to share unexpected and precious gifts from their experience-filled lives.*

Virginia Bell, M.S.W.
Program Consultant, Lexington/Bluegrass Alzheimer's Association, and
co-author, *The Best Friends Approach to Alzheimer's Care*

*This exciting new resource challenges readers to think differently about people with dementia and ways to care. The authors provide thoughtful direction on how to shape care and programs to focus each person's abilities. They remind us to take into account the whole person and to structure care and approaches to reflect that totality. Rather than telling us how or providing "cook book" approaches, they help us find the answers within ourselves and our programs. This is a wonderful new reference for families and professionals alike.*

David Lindeman, Ph.D.
Rush Institute on Aging

*In an extraordinary blend of thoughtful inquiry, philosophical reflection, and hands-on practical guidance, the authors offer a compelling and deeply encouraging framework for restoring dignity, relationships, and hope to persons with Alzheimer's disease and to those entrusted with their care.*

Lisa Snyder, L.C.S.W.
Alzheimer's Disease Research Center, La Jolla, California

*This wonderful book by Sam Fazio, Dorothy Seman, and Jane Stansell offers exceptional insights about caring for victims of Alzheimer's disease. This trio of professional caregivers has extensive experience in caring for persons with Alzheimer's disease in the daycare setting. Their patients have ranged from the mildest to the most severe. Both family members and professionals will benefit greatly by their experience, wisdom and advice.*

Jacob H. Fox, M.D.
Professor and Chair, Department of Neurological Sciences
Rush-Presbyterian-St. Luke's Medical Center

# Rethinking Alzheimer's Care

# Rethinking

# Alzheimer's

# Care

Sam Fazio, Dorothy Seman, & Jane Stansell

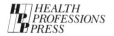

HEALTH
PROFESSIONS
PRESS

Baltimore • London • Winnipeg • Sydney

Health Professions Press, Inc.
Post Office Box 10624
Baltimore, Maryland 21285-0624

www.healthpropress.com

Copyright © 1999 by Health Professions Press, Inc.
All rights reserved.

Typeset by Barton Matheson Willse & Worthington, Baltimore, Maryland.
Printed in the United States of America by
  Versa Press, Inc., East Peoria, Illinois.
Cover by Nancy Johnston. Cover photograph of Jeff Caldwell and Nancy Arendt by
  Bill Richert.

**Library of Congress Cataloging-in-Publication Data**
Fazio, Sam.
   Rethinking Alzheimer's care / Sam Fazio, Dorothy Seman, & Jane Stansell.
   p.  cm.
   Includes bibliographical references and index.
   ISBN 1-878812-62-9
   1. Alzheimer's disease—Patients—Long-term care.  I. Seman, Dorothy.  II.
Stansell, Jane.  III. Title.
RC523.F39  1999
362.1′96831—dc21
                                                                    99-41163
                                                                        CIP

# Contents

# About the Authors

**Sam Fazio, M.A.**, is the Director of Education and Training at the national Alzheimer's Association, where he manages a team that coordinates the development and delivery of education and training programs, conferences, and educational materials. He holds a master's degree in gerontology from Northeastern Illinois University. He has a broad range of dementia experience, including direct care, working with families, professional training, national and international presentations, and publications.

**Dorothy Seman, R.N., M.S., N.H.A.**, has been active in the health care field for more than 30 years. Her practice has allowed her to work with people with dementia and caregivers in many roles such as administrator, educator, consultant, and clinician, and in diverse settings such as hospitals, residential programs, in-home hospice, and adult day services. Ms. Seman has been Clinical Coordinator of the Alzheimer's Family Care Center, an award-winning dementia-specific adult day center in Chicago, since 1989. She works for the center through the VA Chicago Health Care System. Seman also is adjunct clinical faculty in the Department of Medical-Surgical Nursing at the University of Illinois. Ms. Seman holds degrees from Northwestern University and the University of Illinois. She has delivered presentations internationally.

**Jane Stansell, R.N., M.S.N.**, is the Director of the Alzheimer's Family Care Center in Chicago. Ms. Stansell has been a strong advocate for change in the way that care is provided to people with Alzheimer's disease. Her nursing, administrative, and direct care experiences have convinced her that care for people with dementia must support them both emotionally and functionally throughout the illness. Stansell works with other adult day service providers in Illinois and the Illinois Department on Aging to provide consistent educational opportunities for care providers and to develop legislation and administrative rules that meet the needs of people with dementia and their caregivers. She also works with the National Adult Day Services Association to create appropriate outcomes of care for people with dementia and to provide educational opportunities for adult day services providers.

The **Alzheimer's Association** is the only national voluntary organization that is dedicated to conquering Alzheimer's disease through research and to providing information and support to people with Alzheimer's disease, their families, and caregivers.

Founded in 1980 by family caregivers, the Alzheimer's Association has more than 200 chapters nationwide providing programs and services to assist Alzheimer families in their communities. The association is the leading funding source for Alzheimer's disease research after the U.S. government.

The Alzheimer's Association provides information on Alzheimer's disease, current research, caregiving techniques, and assistance for caregivers. For more information or to locate the chapter nearest you, contact the national office at 919 North Michigan Avenue, Suite 1000, Chicago, IL 60611-1676. Telephone (800) 272-3900, TDD (312) 335-8882. Internet—http://www.alz.org. Email—info@alz.org.

For more than 150 years, **Rush-Presbyterian-St. Luke's Medical Center** has been a leader in health care in Chicago and the Midwest. The Medical Center includes Rush University, Presbyterian-St. Luke's Hospital, and the Johnston R. Bowman Center for the Elderly. It is home to the seven Rush Institutes, which draw together patient care and research to address major health problems, offering primary health care services and state-of-the-art treatment for arthritis and orthopedic problems, cancer, heart disease, mental illness, diseases associated with aging, and neurological problems.

The largest private academic medical center in Illinois, Rush is the hub of a comprehensive, cooperative health care system that serves approximately 3 million people in Chicago and its suburbs. The Rush System for Health is one of the largest regional health care provider networks in the area.

The commitment of the medical center to Alzheimer's disease care and research is widely known. In addition to numerous research projects, a variety of programs and services are provided for individuals with Alzheimer's disease and their families. The Alzheimer's Family Care Center was established in 1987 to provide comprehensive adult day services for people with dementia and the family members who care for them.

**The U.S. Department of Veterans Affairs (VA),** Health Care Division, serves the health care needs of U.S. veterans through an integrated system of 172 hospitals and a growing number of community-based clinics. The VA Chicago Health Care System was established in 1996 by integrating the VA Lakeside and VA West Side Medical Centers. The system offers 374 inpatient beds, more than 100 specialty clinics, and 3 community-based outpatient clinics. With greater than 500,000 outpatient visits annually, the system has one of the most active ambulatory care programs within the Department of Veterans Affairs and provides care for more than 40,000 veterans residing in Chicago and the surrounding counties of northeastern Illinois and northwestern Indiana.

# Acknowledgments

We would like to extend a heartfelt thank you to our family, friends, and loved ones for their ongoing patience, confidence, and support, which allowed us to make this book a reality. In addition, we would like to express our gratitude to our employers, the Alzheimer's Association, the U.S. Department of Veterans Affairs, and Rush-Presbyterian-St. Luke's Medical Center, for their support and flexibility throughout the development and completion of this work. Finally, special thanks to Mary Magnus and Health Professions Press for believing in us and providing us the opportunity to share our thoughts and ideas with others.

We also are indebted to the authors and colleagues whose readings and conversations have guided and influenced us throughout our journey. At the same time, we have been fortunate to learn from many devoted families how to reach beyond the dementia to the person. This capacity to focus on what remained and not on what was lost was a beacon that guided our approach to care early on. Most significant, our primary teachers have been the many people with dementia who have shared their unique personhoods with us, often to the very end of their lives. Over the years, these individuals have taught us more about dementia care and ourselves than any article, book, or presentation. We hope to equal their courage, honor their lives, and give shape and voice to a new way of looking at meaningful relationships with men and women who also happen to have Alzheimer's disease or a related dementia.

$\mathcal{J}$ntroduction

As we enter the 21st century, we have seen an explosion of materials on the care of people with Alzheimer's disease. These materials cover a range of topics and attempt to logically describe the disease process and offer simple strategies for care. Although this approach to dementia care education and development has been helpful, for many people these materials are no longer adequate.

Many people want to look at dementia and the way that they provide care differently than we have in the past. Some believe that a paradigm shift is long overdue and necessary to advance dementia care to the next level, which involves perceiving the experience of the disease in different yet genuine ways. This shift requires rethinking much of what we have learned to allow people with dementia to live as fully and richly as possible, not to be defined solely on the basis of their dementia diagnosis. Making this shift involves treating others as we would like to be and deserve to be treated ourselves. It involves putting the *care* back into dementia care.

In reflecting on our own practice and thinking about excellence in staff and the programs that we have seen, most of what has impressed us is not necessarily reflected in the literature. Professional publications provide space for approaches that are based on "bodies of knowledge" and "theories of practice," which are derived from narrowly defined and measured research topics. In practice, however, where many factors influence care, we find that the human element and powerful relationships often are what energize successful programs. In these programs the quality of daily life for people with dementia is greatly enhanced. This human element, or humanity, is the essence of what we consider dementia *care*.

This humanity in dementia care demands something of caregivers: welcoming self-reflection, questioning assumptions, building relationships, and embracing possibilities. Rather than looking only at the person who has been diagnosed, we must look closely at our personal biases, expectations, and contributions. Professionals are rarely, if ever, asked, encouraged, or expected to do this kind of soul searching.

One of the major challenges of reexamining dementia care is adopting an approach that suggests that we set aside our familiar understanding of Alzheimer's disease. To do so, we must consider new or alternative patterns of thinking, doing, and being; we need to jolt ourselves out of a safe, detached approach. At the same time, we must recognize how our very language and way of thinking about dementia has constricted us and limited possibilities.

Many terms have been used so routinely in dementia care that they seem to have lost their precise meaning. We believe that by examining critical concepts such as the meaning of home and caring, by taking another look at our philosophy and the environment, and by exploring new dimensions such as the soul, we can refine our approaches and commitment and revitalize those of others, and together reshape dementia care. This reshaping is actually a "coming home"—a return to dementia *care*.

In a sense, we also experienced a coming home to dementia *care* as we worked together to create this book. Our reviews and discussions allowed us to have an open dialogue about dementia care and our underlying values, beliefs, and experiences. At the same time, we supportively challenged one another to expand our perspectives to recognize other viewpoints. We grew together and became enlightened both personally and professionally. We encourage you to do the same and to share this incredible journey with us.

As you explore each chapter, think through how the ideas presented can be applied within your care setting or to your role. Thought-provoking "Rethinking in Practice" exercises have been included throughout the text to help you find answers or solutions within yourself. You may need to take an honest look at what you think and how you care—including values and beliefs, perceptions, and actions. Done either individually or with others, it can help you unblock old ways of thinking and acting and allow you to discover new ways.

As you read on, clear your mind, open your heart, and embrace the possibilities.

# chapter one

# Reconceptualizing Alzheimer's Disease

*A man traveling across a field encountered a tiger. He fled, the tiger after him. Coming to a precipice, he caught hold of the root of a wild vine and swung himself down over the edge. The tiger sniffed at him from above. Trembling, the man looked down to where, far below, another tiger was waiting to eat him. Only the vine sustained him.*

*Two mice, one white and one black, little by little started to gnaw away the vine. The man saw a luscious strawberry near him. Grasping the vine with one hand, he plucked the strawberry with the other. How sweet it tasted!*

*Reps & Senzaki*

Alzheimer's disease often is characterized by the use of negative descriptors. The language used by families and professionals in discussing dementia includes words such as "inability," "deterioration," "sufferer," "victim," and "burden." Media portrayals of Alzheimer's disease often focus on popular or problematic topics such as poor-quality nursing facility care, aggressive behaviors, or rapid deterioration leading to death. Films and books often are negative and sensationalistic and seem to be designed primarily to attract attention. Often-used titles include "The Living Death," "The Never-Ending Funeral," or "The Burden of Alzheimer's Disease," and the content reflects issues such as coping, controlling, or managing.

This negative focus provides families, other caregivers, and the public with a limited and narrow view of the disease. These negative characterizations seem to contribute to the development of people's perceptions, interpretations, and approaches to care as well as to their overall anticipation and expectation of what lies ahead. People are introduced to and prepared for a grim future filled only with extensive loss and decline. Less negative alternatives to describe Alzheimer's disease must be introduced to families, professionals, and the public. The effects of our descriptions can be monumental; therefore, words used to describe Alzheimer's disease must be chosen carefully and must reflect a more balanced or encompassing view (Fazio, 1996).

**1**

## RECOGNIZING THE IMPACT OF WORDS

Words do shape thoughts and, ultimately, actions. They lead to different perspectives and form a language that has an impact on perceptions. Words come with baggage and possess universal as well as individual meanings, while they shape the consciousness of the people who communicate with them (Gayle, 1989; Muller & Cox Dzurec, 1993). In addition, language and terminology can influence and lead to misconceptions and victimization:

> The daughter of a man with Alzheimer's disease shared her reaction to his recent hospitalization. She described with much frustration how her father was referred to variously as "victim," "vegetable," and "shell." She said, with passion, "I never considered my father a shell of a human being. A shell is something lying in the garbage, like an eggshell. It's something you throw away. You don't love, care for, and respect a shell, but you do a person."

The power of words and language is evident when considering the effects of labeling. Labels become a permanent part of a person and help shape his or her personal and social identity. They dehumanize the individual with the disease while they limit his or her potential and, at times, lead to his or her withdrawing and caregivers' distancing themselves (Goffman, 1963). This dehumanization becomes apparent with Alzheimer's disease as stages, terms, categories, and tests are developed and applied to provide some sort of uniformity to an uncertain disease. Figure 1-1 outlines the effects of labels as well as the possibilities when labels do not exist.

This negativity and terminology is reinforced and fostered by many health care professionals. For instance, they frequently prepare families for "the difficult road ahead" or try to help by suggesting caregiving techniques that manage, control,

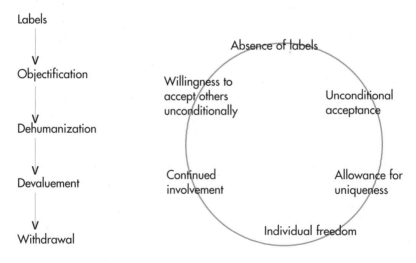

Figure 1-1.   Labeling versus not labeling.

and restrict the person with Alzheimer's disease. Their interventions often can seem one-dimensional, focusing on only the immediate needs of the caregiver. In addition, health care professionals often try to apply a medical structure to an ambiguous, and at times, nonmedical experience.

The stigma of Alzheimer's disease begins with the word "disease." The medical definition of disease has been referred to as a specific entity that is the sum total of the numerous expressions of one or more pathological processes (Cassell, 1991). It is also described as "the professional's construction, perception or inference about a condition with more or less discretely identified characteristics that are believed to be related to lesions and other abnormalities in the structure or function of biological (or psychological) systems" (Wynne, Shields, & Sirkin, 1992, p. 12). Both definitions include pathology or abnormalities that can lead to negative associations. In addition, the word "disease" has come to be associated with impaired health, the constant exploration of causes and cures, and at times, pity—all of which dementia care has enough. Of course the biology of Alzheimer's disease must be recognized, however it does not need to be constantly emphasized or reinforced in everyday care approaches.

The medical model of dementia care, sometimes called the illness model, places emphasis on abnormalities in the structure and function of body organs that lead to disease. The problem is defined as the primary concern. Symptoms are understood to be a direct result of the impairments that are inside the individual's body tissue, and it is assumed that these symptoms are attributed to the dysfunction of the body parts. At the same time, there is a continual effort to outline the stages of disease progression. It is believed that stages are needed to identify a predictable disease course and its associated treatments. However, neither assumption lends itself to the uniqueness of dementia because symptoms often result from factors outside the body, and disease progression is individual. In addition, the terminology used in the medical model often is impersonal, and at times even military-like. Common descriptions can foster adversarial relationships as health care providers discuss wars to be won and diseases to be conquered and defeated. Often, discussions include phrases such as "administering a battery of tests," "identifying the enemy," and "developing a plan of attack." Staffing the medical model are usually a chief of staff, a head nurse on duty, and other charge nurses, who all contribute to a perception of hierarchy, rigidity, and coldness. As you can see, describing dementia in the context of a battlefield is a very defeating framework.

This view of dementia can be considered an example of the "medicalization of deviance," which refers to explaining and treating the person and related social troubles as medical problems (Lyman, 1989). Family matters can instantly become medical matters when someone is diagnosed with a disease. Common characteristics not viewed as problems for individuals who are not diagnosed or labeled with a disease suddenly become behaviors or symptoms that need to be controlled or cured. In some cases every aspect of the disease experience can become over-medicalized or be described in medical terms.

The biomedical view of dementia is narrow and sometimes ignores social forces that affect the definition, production, and progression of dementia. Lyman

(1993) suggests a shift in how the disease is perceived to include a social perspective. This shift includes social factors, nonmedical terminology, and recognition of the individual.

Recognizing the individual is difficult with so much negativity and focus on abnormalities and problems. If an individual is continuously invalidated and objectified, then he or she can lose vital contact with other people (contact with others being considered a significant part of personhood). We must move beyond losses and begin to recognize and support people's strengths and abilities. As one family member said, "He can still do a lot of things if we'd take the time to find them out and then just let him do them the best he can."

The clinical focus, which looks only at problems, also should assess remaining strengths, positive functioning, and individual characteristics (Harrison, 1993). By recognizing strengths and working with the remaining abilities of people with Alzheimer's disease, we can improve the care as well as the experience of the disease. Strengths can be difficult for people to recognize within the context of the existing descriptions of Alzheimer's disease, so we must start this reconceptualization with how we use our words.

## USING NEW WORDS

One way to begin to look at Alzheimer's disease differently is by using different words to describe it. A technique called reframing is used to help people to recog-

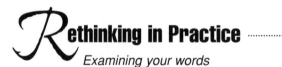

**ethinking in Practice**

*Examining your words*

*Take a look at the words that you use in relation to Alzheimer's disease. Ask others to do the same and discuss these terms. Explore with one another how the words that you use lead to certain perceptions and behaviors. Consider the following questions in your discussions:*

What words do you use to refer to people with Alzheimer's disease?

How do you describe the actions and behaviors of people with Alzheimer's disease?

What words do you commonly read in books and journals or hear on television or in presentations, when dementia is the focus?

What words do you use when talking with family members of people with Alzheimer's disease?

What language do you use when talking with colleagues about people with Alzheimer's disease?

What words do you use in front of people with Alzheimer's disease?

In general, what impact do words have on your thoughts?

In general, how do words affect your perceptions?

In general, how do words influence your actions or behaviors?

nize the positive aspects of situations that were previously viewed as only negative. Reframing has been defined as "thinking about things in a different way; relabeling and redefining behavior, or finding the 'positive connotation' of a behavior or situation" (Pesut, 1991, p. 10). By reframing a symptom, we can understand it as serving a positive function, and, in a sense, every experience and behavior is appropriate given some context, some frame (Bandler & Grinder, 1982; Benson, Long, & Sporakowski, 1992).

Once a situation has been reframed into a more positive context, more choices become available for coping with the challenges that may be involved. When additional options become available, often the tensions and pressures that are associated with seemingly hopeless or burdensome situations are alleviated, and alternatives become apparent (Hulnick & Hulnick, 1989). As words change, so do perceptions, and as perceptions change, so do actions. For example, when the weather forecast tells us that the day will be mostly cloudy, we anticipate a grim day and plan accordingly, but if the day is predicted to be partly sunny rather than mostly cloudy, we interpret the same situation differently. Our changed perception then affects our outlook and how we approach the day. This technique is easily and logically transferable to the experience of Alzheimer's disease to include how we describe the disease, the behaviors of the person with the disease, and our interactions with that individual.

## LOOKING AT BEHAVIORS IN ALZHEIMER'S DISEASE DIFFERENTLY

Many, or all, behaviors that are commonly associated with Alzheimer's disease can be easily reframed to less negative alternatives. Table 1-1 outlines several common

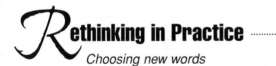

## *R*ethinking in Practice

### Choosing new words

*Think back on some of the words that you and your colleagues identified from the previous exercise. Take a closer look at the words that you use to describe people with Alzheimer's disease and their behaviors. Then think about new words that can say the same thing in a more positive or less negative way. It may be helpful to close your eyes and visualize two different picture frames. The one on the left contains the negative word, and the one on the right is empty: You have the opportunity to create that new word, that new reality. Start with a term that describes the person with Alzheimer's disease. For example, instead of referring to the person as "victim," use "individual." Then try it with a behavior. Instead of calling the person "aggressive," use "energetic." Finally, ask yourself and other colleagues the following questions:*

What impact do these new words have on your thoughts?
How do these new words affect your perception?
How do these new words influence your actions or behaviors?
How can interactions change using these new words?

*Table 1-1.    Reframing behaviors in Alzheimer's disease*

| Symptoms/problem behaviors | Reframed characteristics of individual |
| --- | --- |
| Anxiety | Eagerness |
| Agitation | Energy |
| Wandering | Exploring |
| Pacing | Motivated |
| Decreased attention span | Curious |
| Poor short-term memory | Spontaneous |

negative terms that are associated with Alzheimer's disease and offers less negative or positive alternatives to describe the same words. The left column lists behaviors that are identified as problems associated with or symptoms of Alzheimer's disease; reframed alternatives are suggested in the right column. Common behaviors or characteristics that once were identified with negative actions can be identified less negatively when reframed using different terminology. These behaviors are no longer described as *problems* or *symptoms* but are considered *characteristics* of the person, as they were before the dementia diagnosis was made. By reframing in terms of characteristics, families and other caregivers can begin to perceive and approach these individuals differently, with adaptations, understanding, and solutions. As with any behavior, one must be mindful of any underlying medical cause or preexisting condition. These causes may include chronic conditions (e.g., arthritic pain, fluctuation in blood sugar level) or new conditions (e.g., dehydration, urinary tract infection) and can have a dramatic impact on cognition and behavior. In any case reframing can be useful in helping people to recognize a positive function within a usually negatively described behavior.

As people begin to hear things differently, they can think about things differently and, ultimately, act differently. Reframing provides families and other caregivers with a new way of looking at a situation or experience. It normalizes their experience or situation rather than labels it as something to be treated or dealt with. It becomes something that is understandable, workable, or acceptable. Reframing can be so positive that it is humorous, and thus people may develop their own alternative that fits somewhere between the negative term and the extremely positive reframe.

## TAKING ANOTHER LOOK AT REALITY AND INTERACTION

Thoughts and actions can change as people begin to create new realities using the new descriptions; people make sense out of events and construct their own realities. The same event or situation may have multiple or different realities for different people. The way that we organize an experience, or the frame that we put it into, affects our perception of and approaches to that particular experience (Goffman, 1974). In addition, the way that people construct their beliefs about Alzheimer's disease can affect the way that they manage stress and the way that they care for the person with the disease.

Some people view things differently by looking at solutions rather than only problems. By focusing on solutions, caregivers can identify positive or alternative approaches and adapt or apply them to other challenging situations. At the same time they recognize the opportunities for growth that they can experience. A crisis also can be an opportunity—it all depends on how a person chooses to view it. People possess the ability to create new realities so that different ways of understanding the problem are possible. New descriptions help to create new thought processes. As a family member said, "I used to get so angry when she'd do things and they weren't quite right or the same as they were. It's taken me a while to finally realize that she's trying to help in the best way she can—so what if it's not perfect? As long as I'm open to it, we get along better and things go a lot smoother."

Once negative descriptors are reframed into positive descriptors, new realities can be created by introducing alternative interactions. These interactions also can be described differently, as are the words that are used to describe the person with the disease. Figure 1-2 is a display of the process of viewing an experience or situation as a problem (left) and, alternatively, when it is reframed in a more neutral way, viewing it as a characteristic of the person. Each action is described differently to create an entirely new kind of interaction. The reciprocal loops demonstrate how words lead to perception and perception to action. With explanation and examples of these loops provided, families and other caregivers can begin to understand how their interactions influence and affect outcomes and can learn to focus on solutions. The alternative process helps people to recognize that if something is described and thought about differently, then their actions will be different. Ultimately, interactions can become more positive, successful, and gratifying for everyone involved in the process.

The reciprocal perception process can be easily explained by using agitation and its positive reframe, energy, as an example. When a person's behavior is described as *agitated*, it is viewed as a problem that requires a solution. Caregivers react to the problem, try to correct it, expect the person to do or be responsible for something that he or she cannot accomplish, and try to control the situation that then leads to another problem. When the same behavior is described as *energetic*, it is viewed as a positive characteristic, not something to stop, control, or restrict. We respond to the characteristic, connect with it, accept the behavior or characteristic, and

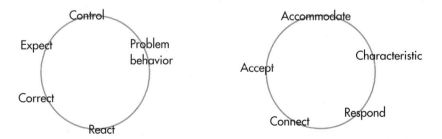

Figure 1-2.   Reciprocal perception process.

accommodate it by finding an outlet for it, such as taking a walk or engaging in another activity.

This reciprocal perception process is applicable to any behavior in Alzheimer's disease and illustrates the results of words, thoughts, and actions. Many times caregivers need suggestions on a behavioral level that can lead to a better conceptual understanding and acceptance on a personal level. Simple alterations can have tremendous, rippling effects not only on care but also on the overall conceptualization of the experience of the disease.

## RECONSIDERING THE OVERALL EXPERIENCE OF ALZHEIMER'S DISEASE

The concept of reframing can be expanded to a much broader context of reconceptualizing, or rethinking, the overall experience of Alzheimer's disease. This kind of reconceptualization can include reframing, a reformulation of the language, and the discovery of positive connotations resulting from the existence of the disease and its associated experiences.

A few authors have briefly addressed issues of reconceptualizing illness and, notably, Alzheimer's disease. Some mention a therapist's positive connotations of Alzheimer's disease on three different levels: individual, familial, and societal (Benson, Long, & Sporakowski, 1992). This concept has been expanded to include

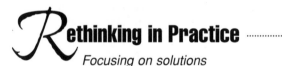

# *R*ethinking in Practice
*Focusing on solutions*

*Think about a problematic situation, but this time do not focus on the negative or problematic aspects of it. Instead, go straight to the solution. Do not add to the problem by reiterating it or making excuses for it; just solve it. Consider the following example as you explore focusing on solutions:*

Each day after lunch, Bill becomes restless and needs to move around. He usually can't stay in the large discussion group with other members, and he often walks the halls looking for something to do. After a while, Bill usually begins tugging at the door, trying to leave the building. The receptionist stops doing her paperwork to bring Bill back to the group activity. The group leader then invites Bill to sit until he needs to leave again. In a matter of minutes, Bill is back at the door wanting to leave. Sometimes Bill gets frustrated that he can't leave and becomes angry or even struggles with the receptionist or other participants.

*What would happen if we switched our focus from trying to keep Bill in the building to assisting Bill in getting out of the building and allowing him to release some of his energy? Think about what might have caused Bill's restlessness or urged him to be "on the go" and then explore solutions. Could Bill participate in a smaller group in the afternoon, take a walk or a ride with someone, or help with yard work? What are other possible solutions?*

the positive experiences that have been identified by individuals with dementia, family members, and other caregivers. Several people have identified the opportunities for positive experiences and natural evolutions and resolutions. Others have described the many opportunities for personal growth and development. Still others describe the various opportunities for deep connections and relationships. The list that follows this paragraph identifies some positive experiences or connotations (Benson et al., 1992). Possibilities for the individual with dementia include the opportunity to live for the moment; appreciate simple things; and accept people without titles, labels, or colors. Families and other caregivers have the opportunity to show that they care, enjoy being together, and can reexperience earlier events with the person with dementia. This concept can only transfer to the community level by promoting awareness of the needs of others as well as awareness and acceptance of individual differences.

### Community Level

Offers opportunity to increase awareness/acceptance of individual differences
Allows for uniqueness
Allows for opportunity to decrease feelings of shame about uniqueness
Provides opportunity to appreciate relationships
Offers opportunity to relate to people on a simpler level
Offers opportunity for community service
Offers opportunity to become less materialistic
Offers opportunity for medical matters to become family matters
Provides opportunity to relate to people on a deeper level

### Dyadic Level

Allows caregiver to share memories/experiences from an earlier time
Challenges caregiver to express caring through adapting
Offers opportunity to express love unconditionally
Offers opportunity to "be" together
Allows for physical and emotional closeness
Offers opportunity for adult child to care for parent
Offers opportunity for surprises/excitement
Offers opportunity to experience nurturing role
Provides opportunity to relate to loved one on a soulful level

### Individual Level

Fosters appreciation for simple things in life
Provides opportunity to live for the moment (ultimate existentialism)
Offers opportunity to accept people for who they are (equalizer)
Offers opportunity to reexperience happy times
Provides opportunity to express feelings and emotions
Offers opportunity not to hold grudges
Offers opportunity to take life lightly (sense of humor)
Provides opportunity to connect soul to soul rather than mind to mind

As words, situations, and experiences are reframed positively, people are able to recognize what Alzheimer's disease gives them rather than only what it takes away. They are able to recognize that when some facets of the individual change, others surface or resurface and allow many opportunities for growth and change. Superficial characteristics that are associated with an intellectual persona may be altered, but the underlying soulfulness of the individual remains constant. The absence of learned personality characteristics can enable the innate soulfulness of the individual to emerge or evolve. Because the individual is unblocked by preconceptions, he or she and family members or caregivers can grow to connect on a deeper level, soul to soul rather than mind to mind.

Petty grievances from the past can become irrelevant as relationships take on a deeper meaning and allow for natural resolutions and evolutions. In a sense people can reconceptualize their experience as a route to more profound, deeper levels of communication. This reconceptualization can be both rewarding and comforting rather than difficult and burdensome, the traditional view of Alzheimer's disease. As the son of a man with Alzheimer's disease said, "It's like my dad was a different man. We got to know each other and related to one another in ways I never thought possible."

## REALIZING THE EFFECTS OF "NEW" WORDS, THOUGHTS, AND ACTIONS

The impact that our descriptive words have is powerful. Our words shape perceptions, experiences, and approaches to care. Less negative or positive alternatives must begin to be used to describe the experience of Alzheimer's disease. The use of these positive alternatives, or reframing, can help people to construct their beliefs based on a more encompassing or balanced view. Families and other caregivers are able to form new approaches to the disease and create new realities when they are introduced to other ways of understanding the experience besides the traditional, largely negative, view. Their approaches to caring for the person are more positive as is their overall experience of the disease. They can begin to recognize the opportunities for growth and personal development rather than focus only on loss, decline, and the "burden" of caregiving. In addition, families and other caregivers can begin to recognize how their actions affect the behaviors of the person with Alzheimer's disease. If they begin to view the disease differently, then their actions can be altered and the experience for the person with the disease also can be different. Individual differences and characteristics can be recognized and accepted. Programs and interactions can acknowledge strengths and abilities and be designed to support them.

Families and other caregivers also are able to have a better experience of the disease when they view it differently. When reframed in a positive light, stressful or troublesome situations are viewed less negatively and at times are perceived as challenging experiences for growth and development. Families can begin to put in perspective their specific situations and realize that the disease experience can have positive aspects and can offer them new and rewarding opportunities. They can choose how to construct their reality and approach their experience. Families and other caregivers can grow to appreciate and embrace certain aspects of the disease experience rather than simply "bear the burden."

The impact of language on perception and behavior is colossal. If people become cognizant of words, thoughts, and behaviors, then Alzheimer's caregiving and family situations may improve dramatically. Individuals must begin to recognize the weight that words carry and how those words shape perceptions, experiences, and approaches to care. Families should not be forced to filter out negativity in order to "survive" and "function." We must rethink the terminology that we use and offer less negative alternatives to the common, dismal descriptors that are used to describe Alzheimer's disease, the individuals who experience it, and our interactions with them. It is only then that Alzheimer's care can evolve and develop into new levels of meaning, thinking, connecting with others, and accepting people for who they are in the moment.

## REFERENCES

Bandler, R., & Grinder, J. (1982). *Reframing.* Moab, UT: Real People Press.

Benson, M.J., Long, J.K., & Sporakowski, M.J. (1992). Teaching psychopathology and the DSM-III-R from a family systems therapy perspective. *Family Relations, 41,* 135–140.

Cassell, E.J. (1991). *The nature of suffering and the goals of medicine.* New York: Oxford University Press.

Fazio, S. (1996, July/August). Rethinking Alzheimer's disease: The impact of words on thoughts and actions. *American Journal of Alzheimer's Disease,* 39–44.

Gayle, J.A. (1989). The effect of terminology on public consciousness related to the HIV epidemic. *AIDS Education and Prevention, 1,* 247–250.

Goffman, E. (1963). *Stigma.* Upper Saddle River, NJ: Prentice-Hall.

Goffman, E. (1974). *Frame analysis.* Boston: Northeastern University Press.

Harrison, C. (1993). Personhood, dementia and the integrity of a life. *Canadian Journal on Aging, 12*(4), 428–440.

Hulnick, M., & Hulnick, R. (1989). Life's challenges: Curse or opportunity? Counseling families of persons with disabilities. *Journal of Counseling & Development, 68,* 166–170.

Lyman, K.A. (1989). Bringing the social back in: A critique of the biomedicalization of dementia. *Gerontologist, 29,* 597–605.

Lyman, K.A. (1993). *Day in, day out with Alzheimer's: Stress in caregiving relationships.* Philadelphia: Temple University Press.

Muller, M.E., & Cox Dzurec, L. (1993). The power of the name. *Advances in Nursing Science, 15*(3), 15–22.

Pesut, D.J. (1991). The art, science and techniques of reframing in psychiatric mental health nursing. *Issues in Mental Health Nursing, 12,* 9–18.

Reps, P., & Senzaki, N. (1998). *Zen flesh zen bones.* Boston: Tuttle Publishing.

Wynne, L.C., Shields, C.G., & Sirkin, M.I. (1992). Illness, family theory and family therapy. *Family Process, 31,* 3–18.

# $\mathcal{R}$evisiting the Concept of Caring

*I knew the nurses by their hands. There was one with such delicate fingers that I cried a little when I heard her come on duty. She made me feel like she had all the time in the world. The others made me feel like a lump of flesh, like they had to get me out of the way as fast as they could . . . But those hands . . . I knew it was going to be a good day when she squeezed my arm in the morning . . . She would put a fresh gown on me and brush my hair with such tenderness and patience . . . You can't imagine how much it meant to me, there in that strange place . . . to be touched like that.*

*Wendy Lustbader*

A concept that is central to the health care professional's (hereafter referred to as "we," "us," or "our") role is providing "care." During its many years of use, this term has acquired some baggage and a number of imprecise meanings. *Care* often refers to the number of people in a census or a particular staff member's assignment (e.g., "We care for 80 people on this floor"; "I'm taking care of seven patients today"). It is a term that often implies a numerical figure, a reflection of workload, and a way of affixing responsibility and determining accountability. In any case, often little attention is given to the fundamental meaning of caring in terms of human relationships. This concept has particular importance in the lives of men and women with dementia. As the disease progresses, they have a greater need for assistance and a decreased capacity for communication and self-advocacy. These radical changes imply that the people providing care assume a greater responsibility in ensuring that they are attuned to the quality of that relationship in the fullest possible way.

In light of the global, progressive, and irreversible nature of memory loss in dementia, the threads of a person's very own identity and his or her coherent connection with others are often strained, frayed, or broken. Relationships are in the "here and now" and therefore carry special importance. Because the self-esteem of a person with dementia can no longer be bolstered by the memory of past accomplishments, the "eternal present" carries great significance.

## CARING FOR A PERSON, NOT A DISEASE

It may be useful to explore our early education and training in the area of caregiving. Most of us were taught to "keep our distance," to "maintain our boundaries," and to "always be aware of our professional role." Usually, these stern warnings were meant to help avoid breaches in professional ethical conduct, to ensure that the provision of care was dispassionate, and to avoid subjective biases in data collection or assessment. These warnings also were issued in hopes of reducing the potential for burnout. The implicit message: Caring can be dangerous to your health.

Another hazard in caregiving is the phenomenon called *identity spread* in the chronic care literature. Often, caregivers tend to relate exclusively or primarily to an individual with an ongoing health condition only in terms of his or her disease. In a sense the person is not engaged as the unique human being he or she is but rather in terms of the disembodied symptoms he or she displays. This objectification diminishes the human potential of the individual and limits the many opportunities to engage him or her on a deeper, more gratifying level. For extended periods and for

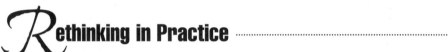

## *R*ethinking in Practice

*Developing awareness and sensitivity about "caring"*

*It is important to develop a common language and understanding of what caring means, in both a personal and a practical way. A useful first step may be to get in touch with the ways we have experienced caring (or the absence of it) in health care and in other settings. This may help each of us become familiar with a way of relating from the inside out. There are a number of ways to help staff develop their awareness and conscious sensitivity to what caring looks and feels like. Think about ways to facilitate this type of learning through staff discussions, role plays, or case examples.*

Can you describe when you or a close member of your family received caring responses from staff in a health care environment or other setting? How did staff express care?

What other encounters have you had where you felt that staff were merely courteous or polite, or where you felt they were just "going by the book" when you hoped for or needed something more? How did that person's response make you feel?

In what way does "caring" differ from "providing care"?

What are some of the ways that you express caring that go beyond "the basics"?

What does caring about or for others feel like to you?

Do you have to like all people with dementia before you can share with them this different type of relating? In other words, do you show caring behaviors toward some individuals but not others?

Do you believe that people with dementia need to experience this deeper level of feeling more than other people do? Why or why not?

In general, how well do you as a care team express this deeper level of concern for the people in your program or care environment?

What do you need to do individually and as a team to increase or deepen the level of care for others?

years into the dementing process, men and women with dementia still respond predictably to human exchanges: responding with warmth to kindness and reacting in negative ways to perceived threats, being ignored, or being overwhelmed by others.

Dr. William Osler, the father of internal medicine, said, "It's important to know what disease the person has, but it's more important to know what person the disease has." By striving to look behind the symptoms to the full human being, we discover many opportunities to connect with the individual in a variety of ways.

## Descriptions of Caring

Several conceptual descriptions of caring can help frame this discussion. The first description is that caring is a moral ideal that rests within a person. This ideal is reflected in one's personal commitment to relate to others in a way that preserves dignity and restores humanity. This way of relating does not make the person feel as though he or she is an object (Watson, 1988). K. M. Swanson defined caring as "a nurturing way of relating to a valued other toward whom one feels a personal sense of commitment and responsibility" (Ryden, 1998, p. 203). It can be useful to explore caring in practical terms, to think through how this concept is expressed in everyday work and life. What do these very common words mean? How do we preserve dignity? How do we relate in a nurturing way with commitment and responsibility? How can a staff member work in a way that does not reduce a person to the status of an object?

## Our Responsibility to Care

In our personal lives, most of us make qualified decisions about who is deserving of our time, attention, and caring. Often, caring is thought about in terms of those individuals who have personal qualities that we like and appreciate. Most people save their deepest caring for parents, grandparents, siblings, spouses/partners, close friends, and children. The norm is to reserve your deepest affection and expressions of caring for "blood relatives" or others invited into your life by your choice, for example, adopted children or long-term friendships. Radiating out from this construct is a second tier of "others" who may include uncles, aunts, and cousins. Another tier might be a group consisting of casual friends or close neighbors. Although differences exist among us about some rules and expectations, it is clear that caring usually is associated with a choice that we make about who is worthy of this gift of our time and our heart. Involved in the decision are qualities of deservedness, likability, and voluntariness.

The type of caring addressed in this chapter makes a different kind of assumption. The expectation is that in a professional capacity, a person is required by a moral code of conduct, by a set of values that is derived from a history and tradition in health care, to treat each individual with unconditional positive regard. The Hippocratic Oath taken by physicians includes the mandate "First, do no harm." Many individuals have come to understand that this mandate includes all health care staff and that it includes not harming any aspect of the full human being—body, mind, or spirit. We should make a distinction between the first kind of caring that we choose to give and a second kind of caring that is what Swanson called "ethical caring," for which there is no precondition or choice based on likability or other criteria. In essence, by virtue of the relationship, a health care provider accepts this expectation of ethical caring.

## Caring Involves More than Providing Care

In the work environment, employers may not be able to require, but the culture should encourage, a deeper level of personal care and commitment that cannot be outlined in any job description. In the course of "assigned work," human beings are at the receiving end of our efforts. In many kinds of care settings with vulnerable older adults, we have much to offer one human being to another. There are many opportunities to provide comfort, share daily joys and sorrows, and interact in authentic ways that acknowledge that the person before us is not only a resident, patient, client, participant, or customer. He or she is much more: a unique individual with his or her own needs and feelings. This person has much to offer and give, if we are open to the possibilities. We can invite a deeper level of involvement that opens doors to a rich and more satisfying relationship that can be mutually beneficial.

In the 1990s and beyond, the focus in health care is on the basics, which often translates to care of the physical being. In the vernacular of health care providers, individuals are assessed by some method that determines their ADL (activities of daily living; e.g., bathing, eating, toileting, walking) status. ADL status refers to the older adult's capacity to perform ADLs. This problem-focused analysis guides staff assignments and the ratio of workers. It is a way of looking that narrows the focus to "tasks," which exclude the critical aspects of the relationship (e.g., choice) that embody the full person. Much of the care that is provided addresses the physical and physiological needs but is inattentive to the quality of the person's life. A Chinese proverb points the way: "If a man has two pennies, he should spend one to buy a loaf of bread to sustain life, and with the other, buy a flower to make life worth living."

## SHIFTING FOCUS FROM CORRECTING TO CONNECTING

Having dementia affects a person's capacity to remember and/or express the specific facts of interpersonal relationships, and whether or how one is related to or knows an individual may be distorted. The majority of people with dementia has a great capacity for gratifying human interactions, however. This capacity can be discovered when others look carefully, are attentive to possibilities, and approach the person in an open, accepting, and giving way. For instance, if a person with dementia hugs you and calls you by her brother's name, it is possible to receive and return this affection—connecting without correcting. Certainly, if the person with dementia is puzzled by the relationship, then you can offer the appropriate clarification, but often the issue

# *R*ethinking in Practice

*Examining ways that we relate*

*It is possible to improve our own skills and to help those with whom we work by demonstrating and talking about the various styles each of us has. We may learn from our mistakes and by watching the way that others relate to people with dementia. It is helpful to think about the many aspects of communication with others. This includes developing an ongoing awareness of what we are thinking and feeling at all times, the various types of body language we use, how that body language affects the person with whom we are communicating, and how his or her responses influence us. Sometimes the environment in which the communication occurs can influence the situation.*

*Select a few situations that staff find particularly challenging. Depending on the comfort level and skill of staff, you may want to role-play one or several recurring events that do not seem to be resolved well. By reenacting such events and reviewing them carefully, staff may be able to discover new ways of understanding, anticipating, preventing, and responding to these events. Looking at these situations as complex events, not just as something that comes "out of the blue," may help us discover many ways to change and influence the process positively.*

*For this experience to be useful, staff must be willing to learn and each member must be willing to share observations, feelings, and suggestions openly. It takes a while to develop this kind of openness and trust, but once these skills are developed among staff, there is tremendous opportunity for building clinical competence, developing broad problem-solving skills, and, ultimately, providing more effective care, with the desired outcomes.*

*Think and share your thoughts about the following situation:*

John forcefully tries to leave the building many times a day. He sometimes curses and tries to shove past anyone who opens or walks through the door. This frustrates John and the staff who work with him daily.

*Use the situation as a role play:*

One staff member can try to reenact how John's scenario plays out each day, and other staff can respond as they usually do. A discussion leader among the staff can then help guide the learning process. Important to focus on is how we can learn better and more effective ways of handling these situations by understanding and connecting with the person, not just enduring the recurring difficult behavior.

*Consider the following questions for discussion:*

How do you think John is feeling? What does he say? What does his behavior tell you?
What are the various feelings John has (as experienced by staff who "play" him) when he is approached by staff who have varying styles?
What goals did staff have in mind when they chose certain ways of communicating?
What are some other ways of approaching John that you have not tried?
When John is not at the door, where is he? What is he doing?
Do you spend as much time trying to engage him as you do reacting to him?
Which times of day are the best for John? Why?
How do you show caring about John in how you respond to him?
Whose needs are you meeting when you react to his behavior rather than respond to his needs?

does not call for clarification. Many times, it is simply a gentle human exchange of comfort in the present.

If our focus is on the quality of our relationship with an individual and not on the particular task to be done as part of daily care, then it is important to evaluate the ways in which we interact with people with Alzheimer's disease in these everyday situations. It is common to see and hear interactions among caregivers (staff and family members) and people with dementia in which the caregiver's language and behavior are focused on correcting the individual. The communication may be characterized by warnings and directives that are filled with many "shoulds" and "don'ts" (e.g., "You should feel better by now"; "Don't go there"; "Don't get up"; "Don't touch that").

Often the facial expression, body language, and tone of voice that accompany these exchanges are firm, abrupt, blunt, or stern, conveying a message of control that may be perceived as quite discomforting, if not outright threatening. It is important for us to develop a capacity to monitor the language and approaches that we use and to be sensitive to how the approach may be perceived by the person with whom we are communicating. It is vital to establish a culture in which colleagues can provide reciprocal feedback about their communication skills. This feedback should include an acknowledgment of skills and abilities, as well as an identification of language and nonverbal styles that could be empathic and nurturing. Many colleagues would appreciate learning approaches that are sensitive and caring, especially in an environment in which both the organization and individuals value learning and personal and professional growth.

When our focus shifts to caring about the person, then the ways that we provide care also need to change. The whole framework of communication will be modified in ways that are positive and affirming when we are connecting without correcting. This change is not merely one of using new words but is actually reconsidering a new approach that puts the person with Alzheimer's disease and our relationship with him or her at the heart of the communication. Instead of saying, "Don't go there" or "Don't touch that," you step back and think about ways to accomplish the same goals without demeaning or diminishing the person. For example, you instead ask, "Could you help me?" or "Would you come this way?" These alternative phrases may help to refocus or distract the person with dementia; at the same time they engage and invite the person and do not demean and control him or her.

Caring is not something that we do apart from our everyday interactions; it is incorporated (or not) into every common human exchange in which we engage. As in the expression "Life is what happens while we're making other plans," caring is what happens while we are involved in the exchanges of daily life. In many work and life situations we get caught up in doing tasks, and we may not be aware of the meaning in the doing. For instance, if we are trying to ensure a confused person's safety by not allowing him or her to leave the building improperly dressed in cold weather, then we can call on many ways to accomplish that task.

Perhaps one reason that communication with people with Alzheimer's disease is not always sensitive or subtle is that often we erroneously assume that the per-

# $\mathscr{R}$ethinking in Practice

*Refocusing and redirecting in ways that preserve dignity*

*Education is not so much filling a bucket, as lighting a fire.*

*William Butler Yeats*

A list of do's and don'ts should be created by each care team based on their particular philosophy of care and values (individual and collective). Rather than teach a laundry list of staff behaviors that are "good" or "bad," it is more important that there be a dialogue about the principles that underpin staff approaches. The act of creating "your way" of doing things gives life to such approaches. It is the process of discussing these things among staff that builds personal commitment, ownership, and shared belief in these approaches. Real learning is in the process of creating, not in the end product itself (lists of do's and don'ts).

A useful exercise for staff may be to discuss their shared beliefs and values and the approaches that are consistent or inconsistent with them. What staff behaviors express those beliefs and values? What other approaches contradict those beliefs and values? It is important not to restrict our responses. Knowing the person with dementia as an individual guides our approaches. What may work with one person and be consistent with his or her personality, needs, and abilities may not work with another. The real art is selecting from various reasonable approaches that are based on the staff's knowledge of an individual. The art and skill in carrying out these approaches effectively involve a lot of focused sincerity. Try to determine why one or several staff members almost always can redirect successfully and others rarely can. Carefully observe what they do that makes this approach work. For instance, is it their timing, body language, tone of voice, desire to succeed, or distaste for power struggles?

*Consider the following scenario for discussion:*

Roy leaves the building with a great sense of purpose. He does not have a coat on, and the temperature is about 20°. It has begun to snow. Roy's balance is poor due to the multiple strokes he has experienced recently. In addition, he has asthma and quickly becomes short of breath when exposed to temperature extremes.

*Ask the following questions to engage discussion:*

What approaches are consistent or inconsistent with your beliefs and values?
Why does it matter whether you use one approach rather than another?
What are you trying to accomplish in this situation?
What are the strengths and drawbacks in using each of these approaches?

*Examine the following approaches that are consistent with beliefs and values:*

"Would you let me walk with you? Would you come with me while I get my coat?"
"Could we have some hot chocolate before we go? I just made some in the kitchen."
"Let's check the weather report before we leave. Please come with me."
"Let me get my car keys and I'll be happy to drive you."

*Examine the following approaches that are not consistent with beliefs and values:*

"You can't go out by yourself, you know that. How long have you been here?"
"The doctor won't let you go off alone."
"Can't you see the weather's bad?"
"We'll go out some other time."

son is not entitled to the normal courtesies of adult communication, the person is not aware of different approaches to communication, or the person no longer experiences emotions. Clinical experience tells us a different story; it gives us a different view of reality. If we are attuned to the ways in which others receive our communication, then we can understand that what we say and how we say it make an enormous and important difference to others. The best evidence comes from the men and women with dementia whose responses to different approaches are available to us if we observe attentively, ask questions, and actively listen to the answers. For instance, when asked how staff could be more helpful to people with dementia, a woman with Alzheimer's disease said, "There are ways to help that don't embarrass you. Use those ways. They feel better to the person." In another example, a staff member in a nursing facility called down the hall to another, "I'm taking Bette to the bathroom to change her diaper." Bette was overheard saying softly to no one in particular, "Oh, you don't have to say that out loud to everybody about me. It's so embarrassing."

Staff learned something from Bette's unexpected revelation—the importance of caring *about* her, not just caring *for* her (personal hygiene/toileting). They changed their thinking, understanding, and behavior because of this experience. Staff no longer called out to a co-worker about the personal care needs of a resident. The staff member's uncaring remark not only hurt Bette's feelings but also conveyed a certain uncaring message to other men and women with dementia who were present. In the course of everyday activities we need to be mindful of using ways that convey active support of the individual's dignity and humanity, so that the person does not feel objectified. In this situation, initially, staff members were not thinking about the feelings of the person whose adult incontinence pad needed to be changed, just the task.

## BENEFITTING FROM CARING APPROACHES

In providing caring interactions and approaches we accomplish a number of things; however, withholding care leads to a different set of consequences. In health care we think about the potential side effects of different kinds of treatments, especially medications. We take this information into account for particular drugs, carefully weighing the potential benefits against the risks. Rarely do we think about psychosocial care in this way or the benefits and side effects of various approaches to daily care. Each individual not only has varied responses to medications based on his or her unique physical characteristics but also has a wide range of responses to various approaches to care.

It is useful to keep this broad perspective in mind when evaluating the range of possible approaches that are available to each of us and to be sensitive to the benefits and side effects that could result from our choices. The term *meta-communication* refers to the great number of subtle messages that are embedded in a particular bit of communication that may seem simple but carry a vast subtext of complex meanings (Nierenberg & Calero, 1978). Becoming sensitive to these nuances in communication can make a difference in the effectiveness and feelings surrounding these daily exchanges.

In many health care settings we hear one colleague say to another, "I can never get him [her] to _____ and you always can. He [she] likes you better." We may know staff members who frequently are involved in events with clients or residents who exhibit aggressive behaviors, as well as staff who never or rarely have this experience. It is likely that although each staff member has a goal in mind, one person has developed a style and approach that is more skillful, based on his or her sensitivity to the approach and a capacity to adapt this approach to each person. For example, two staff members may have the same goal of assisting the person with dementia in taking his or her clothes off before a bath. One staff member may have a secondary goal in mind: to help the individual take off his or her clothes in such a way that he or she is not embarrassed or made unduly anxious. To do so, the staff mem-

# $\mathcal{R}$ethinking in Practice

### Exploring characteristics of caring behaviors and approaches

*The following examples of approaches convey caring along with care. Using specific individuals in your care environment for discussion, consider how well your team measures up to the characteristics below. At the conclusion of the exercise, discuss the advantages and disadvantages of staff members' caring approaches. What is in it for staff? For the people they care for? If caring approaches are good, what are the barriers to providing them?*

Reflects a conscious choice to approach the person as the unique individual that he or she is, offering the kind of intervention that is consistent with the person's needs (e.g., humor, support)

Displays a genuine affection or respect for the person in ways that the person is able to tolerate (e.g., for those who can accept touch, it is shared; for those who cannot accept it, other ways are found to express caring appropriately)

Allows sufficient time for the person to register what is being asked of him or her before proceeding to the next step

Tries whenever possible to use approaches that preserve choice for the person

Does not provide personal care in public places

Understands what dignity means to each person, based on knowledge of and experience with that person, and is sensitive to using approaches that fit the individual

Does not engage in power struggles, is willing to come back later if the interaction is not working, or engages the assistance of someone who may "click" with the person

Interacts with that person, even when a task does not require it

Often goes out of his or her way to do small things that provide comfort or pleasure to the person

Shares information or feelings that go beyond the task at hand, as much as the person can tolerate (e.g., using humorous exchanges, sharing family photographs)

Tries to learn ways to improve his or her skills from the person's feedback and responses

Evaluates his or her role in communication that is not working

ber must be attentive to the feedback he or she receives from the individual and must be willing and able to adjust his or her style according to how the situation progresses.

Often, the difference in how we communicate has at its foundation a conscious decision about how to approach the person with Alzheimer's disease or a related dementia. Some may choose to understand the approach as a task to be done *to* a person, whereas others may perceive the person first as a full human being with feelings and needs that go beyond the task. To accomplish the task, then, we must first try to understand the person and select an approach that is the most beneficial and the least harmful, as illustrated in the following list. The effects of such approaches to care are

- They support self-esteem
- They diminish anxiety and fear
- They help the individual feel safe physically and emotionally
- They let the person know that he or she is cared for
- They support the highest level of functioning of which the person is capable
- They increase the likelihood of successful and timely completion of activity/task
- They provide staff with a feeling of satisfaction and gratification

There are side effects to uncaring approaches:

- Diminished feelings of self-worth
- Provoked fear, anxiety, and anger
- Withdrawal, depression, and aggressive behavior
- Limited capacity of the individual to cooperate
- Extended time needed to complete any task or activity
- Avoidance of the individual
- Burnout of staff members

## PROMOTING CARING ACROSS CARE ENVIRONMENTS

Fundamental values and expectations are inherent in the roles that we assumed when we made the decision to work in health care, regardless of the particular setting in which we practice. The ways in which we are able to express or translate this caring, however, vary with the unique circumstances of the places where care is provided.

Many of the traditional ways in which health care staff and environments have functioned have changed rapidly during the 1990s. This momentum suggests that these changes will continue to take place in response to the desires of consumers, expectations of payers and regulators, impact of demographics, pressure of budgets, and competition between providers of various kinds of services. One of our primary responsibilities will be to ensure that the fundamental value of caring and caring approaches continues to take high priority amidst reorganizations and emerging programs and facilities. Caring is not the same as being professional, polite, friendly, or other terms that convey a temperament or façade of superficial good cheer. Real caring arises from a state of mind and heart that goes much deeper than good cheer. It starts with a personal orientation to others but also demands the requisite dementia knowledge and skills and a depth of understanding about the person receiving care.

During times of rapid and unprecedented changes in health care, staff must have a clear philosophy of caring so that they can understand how they can preserve a caring approach while providing care. Staff members must be able to describe in practical ways how to preserve a fundamentally caring approach, although the way that this is done also must evolve.

In the context of research in a different health care population, K. M. Swanson defined caring as "a nurturing way of relating to a valued other towards whom one feels a personal sense of commitment and responsibility" (Ryden, 1998, p. 203). She discussed five key processes that were observed in her qualitative research that describe caring in ways that demonstrate its practical expression. These processes can show us a way of understanding how this kind of caring can be provided for people with Alzheimer's disease and related dementias across all care environments. Ryden (1998) first described the possibility of adapting Swanson's approach for people with dementia. The following is a paraphrase of Swanson's five processes that illustrate caring in practice:

1. **Maintaining belief**: conveying that the individual has the capacity to survive events or transitions and face a future with meaning
2. **Knowing**: trying to understand an event as it has meaning in the life of the person
3. **Being with**: conveying the feeling of being emotionally present to the person
4. **Doing for**: giving assistance to the individual in the performance of those activities that the person would perform unaided if he or she had the necessary strength, will, or knowledge to do so
5. **Enabling**: facilitating the person's passage through life transitions and unfamiliar events

In the care of other populations, the approach that staff use is often tempered or influenced by the clear responses of the recipient of care. The recipient's feedback helps to shape current and future interactions. In working with men and women with a progressive and irreversible dementia, the feedback may not be verbalized, or it may be somewhat ambiguous. The communication difficulties and unique vulnerability of older adults with dementia make it imperative that staff be particularly sensitive to the impact of their approach on the well-being of the individual and the effects of particular approaches. We must be willing to evaluate the impact of our interventions as a way of evaluating how to improve our practice and care.

## Maintaining Belief

One of the most frequent reactions to hearing a diagnosis of dementia has been a pervasive sense of futility and negativism. The notion of therapeutic nihilism, the view that nothing can be done, is widespread. This negativity has resulted in a common view that having this disease is "a fate worse than death." Lacking a cure and fearing progressive decline, family or friends often say, "If I get like that, just shoot me." One gets a sense from reflections in the lay literature that life with dementia is not worth very much, and it may not even be worth living. Perhaps because we are influenced by the larger culture in which we live, many health care staff may not invest time and energy in the care of individuals with dementia.

A kind of psychological triage process may relegate people with dementia to the category of hopeless/helpless. We may believe (incorrectly) that people with dementia are unaware of our ministering, so we avoid contact or have only minimal contact. This view may indeed relegate the care of people with dementia to a kind of second-class status. Because we assume that our efforts will not change the outcome, we also assume that our care does not have meaning for the person or for ourselves.

Across all care environments, it is essential that we maintain an openness to learning from the person with dementia and his or her family caregivers, and to finding out what activities and ways of relating still hold meaning for that person. Sometimes the capacity of a diagnosed individual to experience meaning in life is obscured by hospitalization, relocation, concurrent illnesses, or sensory overload caused by excess stimulation and unfamiliar environments. Because dementia impairs the capacity of the person to adjust to transitions, we must initiate and maintain the effort to minimize trauma. At the same time our provision of care should guide us in a climate that enables the person to experience, as much as possible, a meaningful daily life.

We must strive to use the perspective of the diagnosed individual to find out what is meaningful to him or her. We must refrain from imposing our view of a meaningful life on the person and strive to understand meaning in a very personal and individual way. One approach is to ask family members what their relative finds gratifying and augment the questioning with the collective observations and assessments of involved staff. Staff must convey through their words and behavior that, despite the individual's difficulties or limitations, he or she will be assisted in staying engaged in life. We may offer words of encouragement, a shared smile at a mistake, or an encouraging hug. Other people with dementia may need direct staff assistance to complete an activity that is progressively difficult. For many individuals with changing skills, staff who can facilitate ordinary activities by providing subtle, timely support are the key to continuity of the lifelong positive sense of self.

## Knowing

Although "doing for" is an important component in caring, caregivers of people with Alzheimer's disease must be vigilant about not overdoing. This is important because of the nature of the disease and the need to reinforce remaining strengths and abilities. One area that has not received the attention it deserves is our lack of knowing who the person is for whom we are caring. What are the unique feelings, wishes, and needs of that person, beyond what we think is helpful? Who is the person as an individual? These men and women are not defined by their disease. They are multidimensional individuals with unique histories, each with a set of human experiences that form his or her identity. To engage them only on the level of tasks to be completed means that we miss a vital opportunity to know one another as complex human beings, with many chances to exchange on a deeper level. It is necessary to expand our way of knowing by moving beyond traditional "assessments." This deeper way of knowing is sensitive to their histories and to their responses to their histories—the meaning that these events have in their lives.

We also can expand our knowing a person by heightening awareness in the here and now. We sometimes lose our attentiveness and miss the opportunity to learn from the many nuances and subtleties that are part of everyday interactions. By consciously trying to be open to learning and paying complete attention to all interactions and observations, we can expand our knowledge about each person in the most fundamental sense, that is, how the individual is most familiar and comfortable in relating to others.

The care of individuals with dementia often focuses on behavior management, with an emphasis on encouraging them to do or not do certain things (e.g., stay in bed at night, eat lunch, change clothing, stay on the unit, stop shouting). Such goals are related to a care plan, or a way of meeting certain health care goals. Many times, we handle them on the surface, attempting to persuade individuals with dementia to conform their behavior to our needs, wishes, or plans for them. This type of communication is one way: We want them to understand and act on our directions or instructions. Our goals may be thwarted if we communicate only in this one dimension. Since the late 1980s we have learned many communication strategies that work to accomplish these tasks. These are useful techniques and strategies, but they constitute only one piece of the puzzle. The other piece requires us to know the needs and wishes of people with dementia for whom we care.

## "Being With"

If we think of our relationship only as one of providing help with tasks, then we miss the chance to relate on a deeper level to other human beings. As in any relationship, we see many possibilities and make specific choices about how much we want to give and receive. With dementia, there are many losses, but not all of them are immediate or inevitable. The losses may result from the conscious or inadvertent withdrawal of affection or spontaneous human exchanges (e.g., affectionate touch, smile). The literature does not include much material about the nonmedical effects of dementia, the more subjective experiences of loneliness, isolation, and the feeling of diminished self-worth. With the increasing emphasis on value-added contacts in Western societies, many people with dementia feel that they are a burden on others. By responding in authentic human ways, we can bridge the gulf of separation created by the effects of dementia.

We can convey the spontaneous communication of being with when we express our recognition and acknowledgment of another human being. Emotional availability can be conveyed by not rushing through physical care tasks or by chance encounters in the course of sharing the same environment (e.g., touching someone affectionately when helping him or her on with a coat, if that is something that you know will elicit a positive response). Sometimes we see or hear the expression of powerful human emotions go unanswered. Although we may not be able to understand and meet the need, we must continue to try. Often, being with is expressed in staff behavior that is conveyed in body language that demonstrates caring and concern. Turning a deaf ear to these plaintive sounds conveys the absence of being with.

## "Doing For"

When efficiency is a highly valued goal, staff must be vigilant to ensure that they do not rush through ADLs in an effort to "get things done" and therefore end up doing for an individual what he or she could do independently. In people with advanced dementia, skills can be readily lost through disuse, even in the brief span of a few days or weeks in an acute care facility or a rehabilitation center. The danger of learned helplessness can be minimized if staff limit doing for only when various strategies for cueing no longer work. Some individuals may not learn to feel helpless but may fall into a pattern of learned dependence, if their self-directed actions are not supported or are consistently discouraged. Approaches that may foster dependence may include comments such as, "I told you not to get up unless I'm there. You're going to fall!" or "I told you not to pour the coffee. You always spill it!"

There are other circumstances in which a limited amount of doing for can facilitate independence in the remaining aspects of care. For example, unwrapping or cutting food for those who need this type of assistance can be a clear way of expressing caring for the purpose of supporting autonomy. Skillful dementia care is the foundation of expressing caring. Caring alone is necessary but insufficient. We must strive to develop ways of expressing caring throughout skillful clinical practice.

## Enabling

In the name of expedience, efficiency, or the prevention of harm, many staff members discourage a person with dementia from using retained skills by not providing the right amount of support at the right time and consistently. Some key functions that staff must attend to include using the bathroom, walking, and feeding oneself, based on the amount of adaptation that is needed by an individual.

Caring, in this most empathic sense, is closely related to providing good care, but it is not the same thing. Employing staff who possess a basic knowledge of dementia and have the associated skills is necessary but insufficient. By understanding the complex individual effects of the dementing illness, staff often can complete care tasks more smoothly and may not have to handle what they may perceive as difficult behaviors. Caring for older people with dementia raises the quality of the interactions to a different level. Staff are able to look beyond their caregiving role, and they are invited to relate more fully as human beings. This deeper level of caring results from staff being able to broaden their relationship beyond completing tasks, which involves conscious reflection about the nature of the relationship and a personal decision to adopt approaches that are nurturing. The new relationship also is based on mutuality and not on a defined unidirectional relationship of one who cares and one who receives care.

Because of their lack of experience with respectful caring relationships, some staff members may not be able to relate on a deep level. There are many ways, however, that a caring team can model this deeper way of relating to people with dementia. In addition, staff in dementia programs must be able to show a level of caring for and about one another as human beings. Providing daily care for people with Alzheimer's disease or a related dementia, although very rewarding, can be depleting. We cannot expect staff to give what they do not feel and experience themselves. Staff must be viewed and treated as multidimensional human beings, not just workers. The culture across all care environments must invite, encourage, and honor this deeper way of appreciating human relationships in the course of daily work. Mentoring programs can be developed to help staff learn the subtle ways that personal caring can be conveyed in daily communication and contact. Caring approaches should be given equal weight and value with the performance of other job responsibilities. Observations of this deeper way of relating should be acknowledged and celebrated, both publically and privately. The decline or death of a client or resident may provide an opportunity to talk about the meaning that someone has had in our work and our life. In these planned and unplanned ways leadership and staff can nurture the many gratifying interactions that are available in working with people with dementia.

The caring way of relating is expressed differently by each staff member, but there are certain characteristics that are evident in any relationship that has great depth. These qualities include an enduring belief that no matter what behaviors or kinds of communication are evident, the person is still a human being, and caregivers must relate accordingly. Each staff member does what is necessary to know this person as fully as possible, including looking beyond the disease. Staff may be involved in completing tasks, in relation to their individual responsibilities, but the relationship is not confined to that. The staff member focuses on being with the individual with dementia in any way that is necessary at any given time. How the staff member is present with the person depends on the situation. Always the focus is on supporting abilities and meeting needs. Being present is accomplished, in very limited ways, through doing things for the person. It usually involves supporting the individual to be as independent as possible, enabling him or her to do whatever his or her capacity allows. This enabling covers all human interactions and possibilities, not solely physical care tasks. It means exploring and expressing feelings and relating and contributing to others.

## CARING INVOLVES LISTENING FOR MEANING

Many of us get caught up in difficult situations and gloss over our successes. Often, the quietly spoken comments of people with dementia go unheard or go unshared with the rest of the staff. Different kinds of feedback can tell us whether we are doing well or need to improve, or both. Keeping a log or journal of comments from notable individuals in your care environment can be helpful. Sharing their comments with others is a way to express pride in your collective successes. An individual may say something that needs to be understood but that takes a bit of discussion to determine its meaning. Because of the short-term memory loss that is associated with dementia, these comments often are gifts to be unwrapped in the moment. Even negative comments can help, by giving us an open window into how the person who is receiving care feels about it. Taken together, these comments can help us develop more sensitive and caring approaches.

The success of these approaches can be measured by the verbal and nonverbal feedback from the person receiving care. If staff use as a measure of success only the completion of a task (e.g., number of baths given, number of meals served), they will be unable to see the more tangible results of how the care recipient felt about it. With a greater awareness of facial expression and body language and by "reading between the lines," we often can understand and feel how the person experienced the care. Success must not be limited to tallying what was done but should include how it felt to those receiving the care. By tuning in to the person's feedback, staff often can change their approach to the person, and the experience can feel safe, enjoyable, gratifying, and meaningful for the person with dementia and staff.

Often, comments carry complex meanings that provide insight into the way that individuals are thinking and feeling about their life and what is happening to them. Some comments can help us in understanding their needs and how we can assist them. Many of these comments offer the guidance that is needed to provide the kind of support or care throughout the course of the illness. For instance, "I was so happy when I heard I was coming here. When I heard I was coming here, I felt like dancing!" (translation: I like attending the day center). Or, when being assisted with putting on his jacket in a rather quick manner, a man said, "Who do you think I am—Houdini?" (translation: Slow down, I'm doing the best that I can). And finally, "I'm not living with Alzheimer's; Alzheimer's is living with me" (translation: I'm still in control, not the disease).

## COMMUNICATING CARING IN OUR CAREGIVING

Once we commit to "caring for" and not just "taking care of" people with dementia, we can and must think about ways this attitude can be woven into our daily encounters. This sensitivity requires us to examine the way that we interact throughout the day. It may help to ask ourselves how we would react to the care if the roles were reversed: Would I be satisfied to be on the receiving end of the care I provide? Am I open to really observing and listening and not focused exclusively on my agenda of what needs to be done? Am I flexible enough to change my attitude/behavior if this seems to interfere with rather than support the quality of his or her life? An example follows:

The situation had been heating up for a while. A woman was feeling stressed by her husband's "stubbornness." She says, "Now, that's enough, it's time for bed. You've got to put your pajamas on, now!" There is angry silence, then he says, "Where is it written?" She considers his words and then reconsiders her request/demand for him to change into his pajamas. She says, "Allan, you're right. If you don't want to wear your pajamas, you shouldn't have to." They both had a good laugh. What could have escalated into a negative incident was literally and figuratively put to bed. They both had a good night's sleep. Stepping back, listening, and reevaluating helped restore the issue to its proper perspective. What could have turned into a power struggle was re-

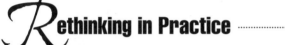

# ethinking in Practice

*Identifying ways people with dementia can serve their community*

*Some programs have had great success in trying to formally involve the people attending their program by soliciting direct input regarding key processes. If staff provide the ongoing structure and necessary support, there can be many opportunities for genuine assistance to members of the program and the community. One of the characteristics of all communities is the willingness of members to contribute to the greater good, often in a volunteer capacity. The time, skills, and wisdom of each member are offered with great pride. It is in the small and large acts of these contributions that one experiences a sense of connectedness and belonging.*

Talk with potential clients or residents about what the program is like.

Discuss their experience in the program with family caregivers, students, and visitors.

Describe how they adjusted to the program, as a way of guiding staff in assisting other individuals in their initial adjustment.

Assist new clients or residents in adjusting through a structured or informal ad hoc buddy system; for example, a familiar face at meals or someone to accompany them to the washroom, as they become used to their new environment.

Talk with staff about the qualities and characteristics that they feel are important in those who work with them.

Participate at some level in hiring direct care staff; for example, incorporate applicants into groups, and allow clients or residents to interact with them in order to elicit verbal and nonverbal responses to applicants.

Involve clients or residents in professional conferences as co-presenters, members of a panel, or respondents to questions about the subjective experience of the illness.

Visit people they know who are in nursing facilities or recuperating at home from an accident or illness.

Share an active role in a funeral or a memorial service for a peer.

Offer information about activities and all other aspects of the program. Are the current activities providing what individuals want and need? Do they have any other concerns about the way that they are treated? Can they offer suggestions to improve their comfort, increase their choice or enjoyment, and so forth?

solved through the wife's respect for her husband's choice in a matter that was important to him. She realized she was being too controlling. She knew that she had no right to intimidate him or try to "boss him around."

Most individuals with dementia seem able to tell us through their words and behavior how we can provide better care and more caring approaches. It can be instructive to involve people with dementia in hiring new staff, orienting visitors, and assisting in the adjustment process of new program participants. A comment from an adult day program participant reflects a common response among her peers about important staff/family attributes: "Tell them it's not so important what's in their heads as what's in their hearts." Other remarks that can help a program or validate efforts include, "I really like coming here. It's really so nice. Everyone helps you, and then we help each other. It makes you feel so good, so happy when you know you're needed and wanted."

## FOSTERING A CARING COMMUNITY

Many varied ways describe the relationship of the members of a dementia care environment. One way is to think of the group as a community, with various members playing a variety of roles over time. In this way of looking at the community, we may indeed think of the members as having a say in how things are run. As part of a community, they are in a position to help newer members adjust and become involved. Many people with dementia have a skill, a willingness, and a desire to contribute in meaningful ways to the maintenance of their community.

If we say that we are serious about a philosophy of care that states that people with dementia are multidimensional human beings who are not defined by their illness, then we are required to reevaluate and rethink many aspects of care. We know that Alzheimer's disease and related dementias are progressive and irreversible and lead to deterioration in many aspects of life. Many individuals who have limited areas of impairment remain on a plateau for extended periods, however. The chronic care literature and the experience of clinicians in many settings is that most individuals yearn to maintain or return to ordinary life, to the simple routines and interactions that are familiar and that give meaning to life. During each individual's journey, opportunities abound to maintain the continuity of lifelong roles and to achieve the satisfaction of giving to others in diverse ways that most have done throughout their lives.

When Mother Teresa was asked by journalists what she thought the greatest work she and others in her order had accomplished through their charitable efforts, she replied, "We don't do great things; we do many small things with great love." This is also the definition, the essence, of the complex caring relationships that many people have in their daily encounters with older men and women diagnosed with dementia. It is this quality that nurtures and sustains both the person with dementia and those who provide his or her care. Alzheimer's disease is not the only or most important factor in defining their ongoing relationship.

## REFERENCES

Lustbader, W. (1991). *Counting on kindness: The dilemmas of dependency.* New York: The Free Press.

Nierenberg, G.I., & Calero, H.H. (1978). *Meta-talk.* New York: Cornerstone Library.

Ryden, M.B. (1998, July/August). A theory of caring and dementia. *American Journal of Alzheimer's Disease*, 203–207.

Watson, J. (1988). *Nursing: Human science and human care.* New York: National League for Nursing.

# $\mathcal{R}$ecreating a Philosophy of Care

*All serious conversations gravitate toward philosophy.*

*Ernest Dimnet*

Most organizations, including health care providers, have a clearly stated mission and philosophy. The mission describes what the organization is trying to accomplish, and the philosophy describes the core values that are believed to be necessary to carry out the mission. Many writers about management emphasize the importance of an organization developing and consistently acting according to a shared set of core values or philosophy (Hammer & Champy, 1993; Jackson & Delehanty, 1995; Peters, 1987). This cohesiveness has been asserted to be critical to the success of any business or service. An effective organization espouses its philosophy and values, which then become a belief system, a culture, or a way of life for those in the organization. This philosophy provides daily guidance for everyone in the organization as they carry out their individual jobs. In no setting is this more important than in one that provides care for people with dementia.

Effectively providing care for people with dementia in a group setting requires that all staff share the values expressed in the organization's philosophy of care. This set of values or philosophy of care must influence every aspect of the organization's operation and care provision, and it must be the basic filter that ideas flow through when decisions are made. It provides guidance in such diverse situations as determining building design or planning outings and provides direction for developing a program, training the staff, and evaluating the program or an employee's effectiveness. When the philosophy of care is shared, it means that each staff member is equally responsible for carrying it out and that there is less need for supervision because everyone shares and lives the same vision and beliefs.

## UNDERSTANDING THE IMPORTANCE OF A PHILOSOPHY OF CARE

Although most care environments for older adults with dementia have a written philosophy of care that emphasizes treating people with dignity and respect, the written philosophy does not always represent values shared by all staff members. Probably no care environment in the world has a philosophy of care that advocates blaming people for their symptoms or treating people in a dehumanizing way, like "a sack of potatoes to be moved from point A to point B," "an empty husk," or "a shell of the real person." Yet, in too many care environments one can observe a person with dementia being led down a hall by the forearm by a staff member with a bored or aggravated look on his or her face. Therefore, although the written philosophy of care is important, it is the values that are actually shared by the staff that have the greatest impact on the actual provision of care.

A philosophy of care needs to be much more than a written statement of beliefs or core values, to be read only by surveyors. For values to be shared universally in any organization, the leadership, formal and informal, must *live* the values that are espoused. All of the staff must see values *lived* by the leadership before they believe them to be important. For others to believe that something is valued, they must see that it really matters. It must be absolutely clear that these values matter significantly to both the formal and informal leaders in the organization and that there is an expectation that all staff will embrace these values.

The philosophy must be talked about often—when problems arise, when things are going well, when someone is interviewed for a position, and when a fam-

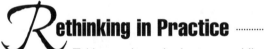

## ethinking in Practice

*Taking a closer look at your philosophy of care*

*It is helpful for each of us to review and rethink his or her philosophy of care periodically. The practice can help keep us focused on what is truly important about what we do. The following questions can be used individually or as a part of a group exercise in reviewing the organization's philosophy of care.*

What core values are described in your philosophy of care?
Do the values described really address the wants and needs of people with dementia?
Are the core values described in the philosophy really shared by all staff members?
Can all staff members clearly describe the core values?
How is the philosophy of care introduced to new staff members? How is "buy-in" achieved?
When is the philosophy of care discussed?
Is the philosophy of care really used as a filter in decision making by both leadership and staff?
Is the philosophy of care specific enough to guide care provision?
What are some recent examples of the philosophy of care in action and some examples when action has been inconsistent with the philosophy?

ily is given a tour of a facility. A philosophy of care is not a one-time announcement, made when the philosophy is written, or something reserved for the marketing staff. When an effective philosophy is lived in the daily details of providing care, it forms a cultural reality and provides a basis for all interactions. When it is determined what beliefs are the core values of the organization, leadership by example is a most effective means of communicating that those beliefs and values matter. The following examples help to stimulate thinking about how a philosophy of care is lived.

If "clients come first" is a part of the facility's philosophy of care, staff need to see this demonstrated all of the time. If an administrator is giving a tour of the facility and a person with dementia is looking for the bathroom, the administrator would excuse him- or herself from the group and take the person to the bathroom. To do otherwise sends the message to staff that "clients come first, when it's personally convenient," and staff very likely will follow the actions, rather than the words, of the administrator.

Because in Western culture "money talks," the budget for an organization provides a clear picture of administrative priorities. The budget is an obvious signal about how much the philosophy of care is valued. Allocating funding to expand administrative staff while cutting funding for activity staff sends a message about the values of the administration. Although there may be valid reasons for this action, these reasons need to be articulated clearly to avoid misinterpretation by staff (e.g., activities are not truly important). Establishing staff performance or evaluation standards that are based on the philosophy of care sends a visible message that the philosophy of care is important to the leadership of the organization and that there is an expectation that all of the staff members will adopt it.

There are a number of benefits for organizations functioning in accordance with a set of commonly shared values or beliefs. Research has found low staff turnover and high morale and performance in such organizations (Dunham & Klafen, 1990). If every employee is empowered to do his or her best work through the shared set of values or philosophy of care, then every experience that people have with the organization will reflect these values. This can have a powerful impact on the feelings that people have about the organization.

## DETERMINING CORE VALUES IN PROVIDING CARE FOR A PERSON WITH ALZHEIMER'S DISEASE

If it is accepted that it is imperative for everyone in an organization to share a philosophy of care, how are the core values that are the underpinnings of the philosophy or belief system determined? People with dementia express the values that are important to them in many ways. Because a primary goal of the provision of care in any environment is to meet the needs of the people in that environment, it is imperative to consider what a person with dementia values and to make those values the basis of a philosophy of care.

## Everyone Should Be Treated with Dignity and Respect

People with dementia retain their basic personality and human spirit throughout the course of the disease. People with dementia, like people who do not have dementia, have a lifetime of experiences that shape their feelings and responses to situations. Perhaps this is the reason that people with dementia say in a variety of ways that they want to be treated with dignity and respect, sometimes in those very words.

A woman with dementia frequently used these words when she told visitors to the adult day center she attended what she liked about the center. When asked what she meant, she often responded that she had been "a tough old bird" all of her life and had always made her own decisions. She said, "Nobody here tells me what to do or when to do it. They respect me and pay attention to me and what I say. It's not just me; everyone here is treated with dignity and respect, so you don't have to worry about what will happen when you get worse." People with dementia who retain good verbal skills are not the only ones who have expressed these feelings, however. An older volunteer who had a habit of calling everyone "kid" said to a person with severe cognitive impairment, "How are you doing, kid?" The person grabbed her arm and said forcefully, "I'm a man."

There is almost universal agreement that all people, including those with dementia, should be treated with dignity and respect. It is nearly impossible to read any material about philosophies of care without reading about treating people with

## *R*ethinking in Practice

*Identifying values in providing care that are important to people with dementia*

*Although it is important for staff to determine what beliefs and values they share, it is equally important to consider whether the values of the staff and of people with dementia are congruent before the philosophy of care is written.*

*It may be helpful to ask people with dementia who have the verbal skills and ability to follow an abstract discussion what is important or helpful to them. Because many people with dementia have some difficulty responding in this way, it also may be helpful to keep a journal listing comments that provide information as to people's feelings about how care is provided. The values that are listed may help staff think about concepts to listen for in interactions with people with dementia.*

Everyone should be treated with dignity and respect.
Relate to the person, not the disease or its symptoms.
Control issues are muted.
Autonomy is more than choices.
Dementia is more than loss and decline—people retain skills.
To facilitate the use of retained skills, one must compensate for losses.
Basic human needs are the same for everyone, including people with dementia.

dignity and respect, but what does it really mean? How is this value *lived* in daily caregiving relationships?

## Relate to the Person, Not the Disease or Its Symptoms

People with dementia want and need relationships that validate them. One man told his wife, "I know I forget things now, but I am most comfortable when people treat me like they always have. I am the same person I always was, even though I have Alzheimer's. It bothers me when I am treated differently." Disability activists mounted a media campaign to change the public's thinking about people with disabilities. One public service announcement emphasized the importance of "treating a person with a disability like a person." Relationships with people with dementia cover much the same continuum as relationships with people who do not have dementia. The primary difference in the continuum is that people who do not have dementia must accommodate the symptoms or compensate for the losses of the person with dementia in order to sustain the connections that are customary in relationships.

To accommodate the symptoms of any illness, the symptoms must be accepted as a part of a disease, not as defining a person. Many people have ongoing health conditions, such as arthritis or diabetes. Writers about these conditions frequently emphasize that people with an ongoing health condition normalize or accommodate the symptoms of the illness and do not always think of or describe themselves as ill (Heiss, 1997). If asked about their illness, their response often is like that of an older woman attending an adult day program: "My arthritis doesn't bother me much, as long as I remember I am an old lady now, and I can't go as fast or as long as I used to." To an objective observer this dynamic woman seemed impaired, although it was clear that she did not think of herself that way and would have strongly resisted being treated as an invalid. Despite this woman's physical impairments, one never would have thought of her primarily as arthritic. Western society has become more sensitive to accepting and accommodating the symptoms of physical disabilities, although the same level of acceptance and accommodation of the symptoms of cognitive disabilities has not occurred. And yet this must take place if we are to move beyond seeing only the symptoms of the disease and come to know the person with the disease.

We also must accept that a person's actions and behaviors have meaning. A widely accepted principle of psychology is that all behavior has meaning (Freud, 1972), yet it is not uncommon to hear the attempts at communication by a person with dementia described as "meaningless repetitions." When verbal communication skills become increasingly impaired because of the disease process, nonverbal communication through actions and behaviors becomes critical to maintaining a relationship. This requires real effort until it is incorporated into our thinking and becomes second nature. The primary importance of this process is the need to accept that the person with dementia is probably not able to change a particular behavior and that we, not the person, must make changes.

## Control Issues Are Muted

Maintaining balance in control issues is essential in relationships. People view control in a situation as positive and lack of control as negative. Lack of control in a situation often leads to anxiety. Because we want to reduce our own anxiety, we want to feel in control of our situation. However, when we exert control at someone else's expense, like Nurse Ratched in Ken Kesey's *One Flew Over the Cuckoo's Nest*, we diminish our ability to have a meaningful relationship with that person.

Because the person with dementia has the same need to be in control of a situation as anyone else, power struggles can result. Power struggles with someone with dementia should be avoided, unless serious issues of safety are involved. As one person with dementia said to a staff member, "When you 'lose it,' we all lose." For example, Gino received a green coat for Christmas. His old one was blue, and he could not remember that this green coat was his, even with his name written in large letters inside the coat. Gino looked for his coat every afternoon when it was time to go home from the adult day center. He went to the closet and put on any blue coat that he found. Getting him out of someone else's coat was difficult, and the need

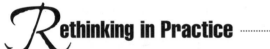

# ethinking in Practice

*Sustaining relationships with people with dementia*

*Compensating for losses while maintaining the essence of relationships that are comfortable and validating for a person with dementia can be challenging but infinitely rewarding. The following examples may help spark thinking about other ways to sustain relationships that are validating and rewarding.*

Ed can still eat finger foods, but he is easily distracted and does not always recognize food on a plate. When staff see him finish half of a sandwich, they can make eye contact, smile, and wait for him to return the smile, then place the other half in his hand. He can then move the sandwich to his mouth independently and continue to eat without assistance until the sandwich is gone. This approach supports his retained skill (getting food into his mouth independently), while avoiding undue distractions and helping maintain a connection with him as a person.

John retains a strong sense of independence, but he needs assistance with wayfinding. Making a comment such as, "Let me show you the way," and escorting him to where he is going compensates for his loss but does little to support his self-esteem. A comment such as, "I'm going to the parlor, too. May I join you?" compensates for his wayfinding difficulty and respects his sense of independence. If a staff member slips her hand under his upper arm, he will straighten his shoulders, extend his elbow, and escort her in a gentlemanly fashion. This small nonverbal recognition of his self-perception as a gentleman is validating to him and helps staff to connect with him as a person, without any extra time or effort.

*It may be helpful to spend some time thinking about other situations and ways to sustain relationships.*

to develop a way to avoid the situation quickly became apparent. After thinking of possible alternatives, staff decided that the simplest thing to do was to move all of the blue coats out of the closet. When Gino did not find a blue coat in the closet, he announced that his son Don had his coat and that he would wait until Don came to the center. Anticipating and preventing problems in such a way often is much easier than solving them after they occur and avoids needless power struggles.

## Autonomy Is More than Choices

Autonomy is a highly valued concept in Western society and an ethical principle much discussed by health care professionals. The Patient Self Determination Act of 1990 (PL 101-508) emphasizes an individual's right to make decisions about his or her health care, and passage of this act formally marked the end of the paternalist era of decision making in health care. One of the primary effects that this act has had in dementia care is to address questions about the decision-making capacity of people with dementia. It is commonly assumed that a person with dementia is unable to make reasonable decisions. Just as there are gradations in the capacity of a person with dementia to do many things, like brushing his or her teeth, there are gradations in the capacity to make decisions. The situation is not simply that the person either has the capacity or does not.

One of the trickiest balances to strike in dementia care involves decision making. Early in the course of the illness, people may have little difficulty making decisions. Even though decision-making skills become impaired as the disease progresses, most people with dementia are able to indicate their preferences. However, as people lose the ability to weigh all of the pros and cons of an issue, they find it impossible to continue to make all of the necessary life decisions. The responsibility to compensate for their losses and support retained skills falls to those who care for them.

Autonomy is the quality or state of being self-governed. Although this definition certainly includes making choices, it encompasses much more. It is feeling in control of one's actions and situation. This feeling of being in control needs to be supported throughout the course of Alzheimer's disease or a related dementia. Supporting the need to be self-governing must be genuine. For instance, "menu choices" alone, like providing the choice between chicken or beef at dinner, will not meet a person's need to be self-governing.

Early in their illness, people with dementia should be given the opportunity to execute a durable power of attorney for health care and to discuss with family and others the kind of care they want at the end of life. A basic premise of hospice care is self-determination, and a person with dementia needs the opportunity to make these wishes known, before the disease process diminishes the ability to do so. Opportunities to execute other legal documents, such as a durable power of attorney for property and a will, should be provided so that people are able to make their wishes known.

In times of need or joy, some people with dementia, like some people who do not have dementia, want to do something for others. To be supportive of this choice, we need to provide the opportunity for them to carry out their generous wishes. This may be done in a variety of ways, depending on the person's retained skills. Making cookies appropriate for a holiday, making gift wrap and wrapping gifts for children in a homeless shelter, or giving a baby shower for a pregnant staff member all are common activities that people with dementia may have the ability and desire to do. Our task is to provide the means and opportunity.

## Dementia Is More than Loss and Decline—People Retain Skills

Traditionally, dementia is associated with loss—of memory, of the ability to do many activities that one has always enjoyed, of the ability to care for oneself, and even of self (Cohen & Eisdorfer, 1986). Although loss certainly is a defining characteristic of all of the dementias, one should never assume that all life skills and feelings are completely lost, as the following example illustrates.

> Before developing Alzheimer's disease, Leo had been an orthopedic surgeon who was committed to helping residents and young surgeons develop their skills. Even in the later stages of the disease, his commitment was evident. Whenever medical students or residents visited the adult day center that he attended, Leo often sat in on their orientation. When asked whether he wanted to add anything during the orientation of a group of medical students, he thought for a while, pointed to his Safe Return bracelet (an Alzheimer's Association program), and said, haltingly, "It says memory loss . . . sometimes it's hard . . . hard to . . . to . . . ." (the word "communicate" was supplied). "Yes, that's it . . . to communicate . . . but you don't lose it all." Leo's simple but powerful words clearly express the feelings of many people with Alzheimer's disease, family members, and professional caregivers: Although there are many losses associated with dementia, people retain many skills and abilities.

Many people define themselves and others by their abilities rather than by the unique human spirit that defines each of us. Defining people in this way creates the bias that people with many abilities or talents are more valuable than people with fewer or diminished abilities. It also encourages dehumanizing individuals with diminished abilities rather than focusing on the skills and abilities that remain.

Retained skills is a critically important topic that is not often discussed in connection with dementia, perhaps because the losses are so much more apparent and distressing for the person with the illness and for his or her family and friends. In a series of features about Alzheimer's disease on a weekly television program a caregiver stated, "My mother can't do anything now. I have to do everything for her." Yet the caregiver's mother was shown eating breakfast without assistance and rolling out dough in a cooking activity at an adult day center. The woman obviously had lost many skills, but with other people helping to compensate for her losses, she was able to use her retained skills. Sometimes we get so caught up in the increasing need to compensate for losses associated with the illness that it is easy to overlook a person's strengths and abilities.

Because some form of the many skills, abilities, attitudes, and feelings developed throughout a lifetime remain, people are not transformed into an "empty husk" or a "shell of the former self" by dementia. This concept is important for many reasons, especially because of the fear that the concept of "an empty mind" conjures in people with the illness. Robert Davis (1989) vividly described his fears of losing his sense of self-worth and even his humanity in the "darkness" of the disease in his book, *My Journey Into Alzheimer's Disease.* The loss of memory or of the ability for self-care does not result in a loss of a person's humanity. Prime health is not a necessary and lasting quality of an individual. What does last is personality and the human spirit, the basis of self-worth—these are retained throughout the course of the disease. It is critical to keep in mind that Alzheimer's disease can last for many years and is progressively degenerative. The loss of skills and abilities is very gradual throughout the course of the illness. Therefore, people have and can use retained skills throughout the course of the illness, as illustrated in Figure 3-1.

The importance of this recognition of people's abilities and contributions cannot be emphasized enough. Because, in general, Alzheimer's disease is thought of by professionals and the public solely in connection with a person's losses and needs, abilities and retained skills are rarely mentioned. In fact, the term *care receiver* is often used in the professional literature to describe people with dementia, implying that they no longer have the capacity to give. This pervasive negative perception can make a diagnosis of dementia or Alzheimer's disease especially painful for both people with the illness and their family members. As one person with Alzheimer's put it, "When they told me what I have, I felt I had been stabbed in the

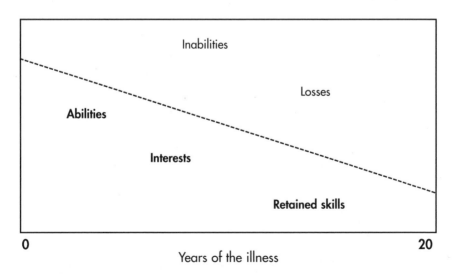

Figure 3-1.   Impact of dementia on a person's skills and abilities.

heart." An emphasis on remaining abilities may help to change the general perception about the disease and reduce the despair that this person experienced.

## To Facilitate the Use of Retained Skills, One Must Compensate for Losses

When we think about people only in terms of loss, we do not look for and support their remaining abilities, which can lead to the development of excess disability or more impairment than the disease process itself causes. As people lose the ability to initiate actions, they may appear to lose the ability to do many tasks. If they are given help to initiate an activity or a task, often they still have the ability to do that task. This process can be compared to jump-starting a car—the battery may not have the capacity to start the engine, but once started, the engine will run.

For example, although Catherine had always been zealous about cleaning her house, she stopped doing this and no longer even vacuumed. It seemed that she

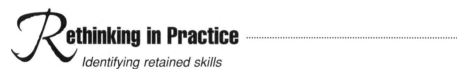

## ethinking in Practice

*Identifying retained skills*

*We must move beyond thinking of people only in terms of their losses before we can readily identify retained skills. We must accept the premise that all life skills are not lost until a person dies. Acceptance of the concept of retained skills frees our thinking, takes our assessment process in a new direction, and gives us an appreciation of people's abilities. We begin to think about what skills and interests this person had before the illness. This is important because not everyone has the same skill set before the illness begins. We need to know what skills the person had and what are his or her habitually used skills. For example, the bookkeeper who added long rows of numbers without a calculator may retain these math skills far into the illness. The person who had exceptional social skills may retain these life patterns long after verbal skills are lost.*

*An effective way to identify retained skills is to learn about the whole person. Select a person and explore the following questions in depth. Describe what changes could be made in care if all staff had this sort of in-depth knowledge.*

What was important to this person throughout life?
    What were this person's passions?
    What brought this person pleasure at work and/or in leisure time?
How did this person respond to challenges and frustrations throughout life?
    What is this person's temperament now?
    What seems to bring this person enjoyment and frustration now?
What is a typical day like for this person?
    Which activities or tasks are most pleasurable? Which are least pleasurable?
    How does he or she enjoy spending the day?
What are the gradations of assistance needed to do a specific task? (For example, can he find the toothbrush and toothpaste, open the toothpaste, put it on the toothbrush?)

had lost the ability to vacuum, but actually she had lost the ability to initiate the task. Vacuuming is often thought of as a singular and simple task. However, if an individual does not know where the vacuum cleaner is, where the electrical outlet is located, or how to turn on the machine, it is an impossible task. When the vacuum cleaner is taken out of the closet, plugged in, and turned on, and Catherine is asked to vacuum the room, she does a thorough job. Conversely, expecting someone with dementia to overcome the symptoms of the disease leads to frustration for the person and those providing care. Many people expect the person with dementia to do something impossible, such as remembering where the bathroom is without environmental cues (e.g., directional signs, an open door so that the toilet is clearly visible) that compensate for losses. Such cues and support must be gauged carefully to meet the person's level of need and not exceed or fall below the amount needed. Too little help could result in failure at the task or activity, and too much help may result in the person's losing retained skills and developing excess disability.

Understanding how the person with dementia experiences the illness and having realistic expectations about his or her functional ability can lead to a realistic understanding of how to accommodate the symptoms of the illness. Most professionals can list the major symptoms of dementia without difficulty (e.g., memory loss, language difficulties, impairment of visuospatial skills, changes in cognition, changes in emotion or personality). However, ways to accommodate these symptoms, so that the person with dementia can use his or her remaining skills, cannot be listed with equal ease. One of the reasons for this difficulty may be that, although there are similarities in the basic symptoms of dementia, there also is great heterogeneity in the range of abilities before a person develops dementia and throughout its course. Family and professional caregivers must accept the responsibility to look for and support the remaining skills of people with dementia.

The need to accommodate the symptoms of a physical illness is well accepted, and there is a long tradition in health care and social services of this accommodation. For example, people with diabetes are provided special diets to accommodate the inability of their bodies to produce the insulin needed to metabolize food. Variation in symptoms among diabetics is expected. Some diabetics need only oral medication and to pay reasonable attention to their diet in order to maintain a safe blood sugar level. Other diabetics need to monitor their blood sugar level several times a day and carefully regulate the amount of insulin to match their bodies' specific metabolism at a specific time. The same sort of acknowledgment and acceptance of gradations is needed in relation to the capacities of people with Alzheimer's disease.

To compensate for the losses of people with dementia, we first must identify the barriers to using retained skills. Some barriers are related to the illness, some are environmental, and, unfortunately, some are created by care providers. In many settings professionals provide care in a way that creates excess disability rather than places emphasis on preventing excess disability by using every retained skill. Part of the reason for this may be because staff in most long-term care settings like to be helpful and believe that if they are not doing something for the person with dementia, then they are not doing their job. Another reason misguided care provision may occur is lack of education about the importance of retained skills and a lack of emphasis on _living_ a philosophy of care that accentuates maximizing the use of these skills.

## Basic Human Needs Are the Same for Everyone, Including People with Dementia

The unique strengths and needs that each of us has are a part of what defines our personality and human spirit. While recognizing this level of individuality, each of us also has some needs in common that must be met in order for us to function successfully, using our unique talents and abilities. Maslow's (1954) description of these basic human needs has long been accepted and often is used as the basis for the provision of health care and social services. These needs include physiological, safety, love and belonging, self-esteem, and self-actualization. These needs are hierarchical, and needs at the foundation of the hierarchy, such as physiological or safety needs, must be met before focusing on higher-order needs.

Meeting the basic human needs of people with dementia is essential in any caregiving situation. Most regulations that concern providing care for people with dementia focus primarily on meeting physiological and safety needs. Although meeting the most basic human needs of people with dementia is essential, it fails to acknowledge the totality of the person. All of us need to be safe from harm and have enough food, water, and so forth, but none of us wants those around us to focus solely on our bodily functions and safety needs. In the novel _Old Friends_, Tracy Kidder (1993) described a character's efforts to change the behavior of a nursing assistant who inquired about his bowel habits in a very public way. The character recognized her need for the information, but he was embarrassed by the way she asked

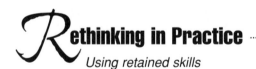

# _R_ethinking in Practice

_Using retained skills_

_The following questions may help in identifying barriers that prevent or make it difficult for a person to use retained skills:_

What do you do that prevents a person from using his or her retained skills?
Do you feed someone because he or she eats too slowly?
Do you button his or her sweater because it is quicker?
What are three alternative actions that would make it possible for the person to do at least part of the task?
What environmental barriers hamper a person in using retained skills?
Does the noise level in the room overstimulate the person?
Are other activities in the room distracting the person?

_It may be helpful to discuss ways to alter where, when, and how care is provided in order to minimize these environmental barriers._

for it and recommended a more sensitive alternative. Focusing only on lower-order needs is a part of the process of dehumanizing people with dementia—reducing them to the most basic needs that are shared with all living animals. This may seem an exaggeration, but how often does one hear a person with dementia described as a "feeder" or "wanderer"?

Another danger of focusing solely on lower-order needs is that early in the Alzheimer's disease process, people are able to meet most physiological and safety needs, which leads many professionals to believe that the person has no unmet needs. This belief is understandable because most "health care" is really "illness care" and is focused primarily on physiological or functional problems. This approach to care may be appropriate for illnesses that have a circumscribed impact on a person (e.g., appendicitis, broken ankle); however, the impact that Alzheimer's disease has on a person is global. Therefore, care for the person with dementia must be focused on the whole person, not just on part of the person. Perhaps one of the major reasons that the medical model of care does not meet the needs of the person with dementia is the lack of attention to higher-order needs such as love and belonging, self-esteem, and self-actualization. More attention must be paid to meeting these higher-order needs.

**Love and Belonging**    All people, including those with dementia, need the opportunity to give and receive affection and enjoy the companionship of others. For this reason caring must be a component of care. The concept of "failure to thrive" was documented many years ago and shed light on the importance of caring in providing care in orphanages (Mitchell, 1977). The children who did not receive affection failed to thrive even though their biological needs were met. This same sort of withdrawal and apathy can be observed in people with dementia in situations in which care is provided in technically correct but uncaring ways. It should not surprise us then that people with dementia become withdrawn and unresponsive if only their biological and safety needs are met without a sense of caring in the relationship (Lubinski, 1991).

Expectations of the person with dementia are a determining factor in a relationship with that person. If one expects that a person's humanity is not defined by good health, then it is not diminished by the losses that are associated with Alzheimer's disease. If one expects that the disease or the symptoms of the disease do not define a person, then the relationship can be based on the person's preferences for interaction. Subscribing to the "empty husk" notion can lead to devaluing and dehumanizing people with dementia and to the inevitable consequences of treating people in a demeaning way—powerlessness, apathy, and withdrawal (Kitwood & Benson, 1995).

People with and without dementia thrive only if they feel a sense of love and belonging. One of the reasons that pet therapy is thought to be effective with people with dementia may be that animals, especially dogs, give unconditional affection. Although pets bring pleasure into many people's lives, the responsibility for meeting the needs of the person to give and receive affection should not be restricted to animals. People with dementia retain a capacity to express and receive affection in ways that can enrich the lives of the people around them.

**Self-Esteem**    Another human need is to experience success. The experience of success is critical to the development or maintenance of a positive self-concept. For people to continue to perceive themselves positively, they need opportunities to be successful. This basic human need is not lost when people are diagnosed with dementia. Two of the frequently voiced fears of people with dementia are "being useless" and "a burden" to others. Structuring an experience to promote success requires thinking differently about the dementia and compensating for losses so that retained skills can be used. The field of psychology has focused much time and energy on how self-esteem is developed and what kinds of input promote or negate its development.

For example, for many years Ann's son stopped by several mornings a week to have breakfast with her. As she became impaired, he increased the frequency of his visits to daily and subtly compensated for her losses: "I'll fix the eggs, and you do the coffee." As her disease progressed, his contributions to fixing their meal increased: "I'll measure the coffee, and you fill the pot with water." He was so successful in subtly compensating for her losses that she never felt incompetent. Even when she was profoundly impaired, she treasured their time together and often talked about how much they both enjoyed visiting while they fixed breakfast together.

In contrast, some people not only are provided meals by others but others place the food in their mouths; these people are even labeled "feeders." When staff are asked why meals are conducted in this way, time and tidiness are often given as

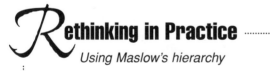

# *R*ethinking in Practice
### *Using Maslow's hierarchy*

*If we accept that people with dementia have the same needs that Maslow described as being basic to all humans, how is that belief lived in providing daily care?*

List the care provided for a particular person that is appropriate for each of the five needs that Maslow identified. Are all of the needs addressed? What changes could be made to more fully address all of the levels of need?

Connect Maslow's hierarchy to Swanson's model of caring described in Chapter 2 ("a nurturing way of relating to a valued other toward whom one feels a personal sense of commitment and responsibility" [Ryden, 1998, p. 203]). If care is provided in ways that help the person maintain belief or meaning in life, does it meet the need that Maslow identified as self-actualization?

Use Maslow's hierarchy to review the monthly activity calendar. What needs are being met by the activities listed?

Considering the hierarchical nature of Maslow's theory, are there ways to organize activities to address these needs more fully?

the reasons: "It takes them too long," or, "They are too messy." Often, the same staff complain about how overwhelmed they are and how difficult it is to feed two or three people at the same time. Being fed as a part of a group of even two or three must be a humiliating experience and leads one to wonder how a person's feeling of competence and appetite would be affected in such a circumstance. Experience in some care environments has demonstrated clearly that even people who are profoundly impaired by dementia can continue to feed themselves if the food is prepared and served in ways that compensate for their losses. This approach has a dual benefit: The person feels more competent and not as many staff are needed to serve meals. Good care also can be cost-effective care.

As people become more impaired, it is imperative to remember that the goal of doing a task is not to complete the task perfectly but for the person with dementia to feel a sense of competence and success that promotes self-esteem. If the person no longer gets the dishes clean when he or she washes them, instead of pointing out this failure we can express appreciation for the help. We can wash the dishes again later, when the person is not in the kitchen. Alternatively, objects can be kept handy just to be washed. For instance, Tupperware can be kept in a cabinet for the person with dementia to wash while lunch is being prepared.

**Self-Actualization**     Maintaining a connection to the community and to other people is important to help meet the human need for fulfillment. The need to make

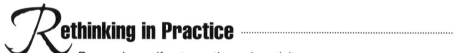

## ethinking in Practice

*Preserving self-esteem through activity*

*Often, a person with dementia wants to help, but he or she no longer has the skills that are necessary to do a particular task. To be consistent with a philosophy of care that mandates being supportive of this desire to help and to provide a task that leads to successful use of specific retained skills, it is helpful to keep activity boxes stocked and readily available. Below are some ways to translate the values in a philosophy into daily care. It may be helpful for staff to explore the creation of activity boxes to utilize specific skills and ways to present the activity or task to enhance the person's self-esteem.*

*The kinds of activity boxes that can be created are seemingly infinite—silver and silver polish, shoes and shoe polish, a jewelry box with assorted costume jewelry, wood and sandpaper, to name a few. Having these activities ready enables staff to introduce an activity at the appropriate moment, rather than lose the moment by having to look for supplies.*

*How the activity is presented to the person with dementia is critical in supporting the person's self-esteem and interest in the activity. A resident might be asked to help clip coupons by saying, "I'm going to the grocery store. Would you please help me clip some coupons? It will help me save some money. Groceries are so expensive these days." Staff could get out a box filled with coupons and scissors, and, after working together for a few minutes, say, "I'll sort these into stacks while you cut them out." After the person is engaged, ask, "Would you mind finishing this stack while I get some coffee for Joe?"*

a contribution and feel that we are doing something worthwhile often is overlooked in the hectic pace of everyday life. A person with Alzheimer's disease clearly expressed this need when she said, "I feel that I have the sword of Damocles hanging over my head, and I need to work hard to make all the contributions I can while I am able." Many people with dementia have expressed the same feeling when asked if they wanted to participate in a research study. One man said, "I want to do anything I can to help them (the researchers) find out more about this disease."

Giving to others is an important value in Western society and is shared by many people. Many of us derive great satisfaction from volunteer work because it is a way to give back to the community. Helping others is a value that is not lost when people are diagnosed with Alzheimer's disease or a related dementia. They need the opportunity to give, not just receive. The kinds of contributions that can be made depend on their retained skills and their wish to be involved in the community, however that is defined.

People with many retained skills may be able to contribute to the community by participating in a variety of volunteer projects. Participants in an early-stage Alzheimer's disease program at an adult day center do volunteer work that ranges from helping nonprofit organizations such as the Red Cross with mailings to caring for preschoolers while mothers in an abused women's shelter meet in a support group. One person with dementia who could read and had a resonant reading voice made tapes for the blind. The contribution may be tangible work, assistance or encouragement to another person, or simply a smile.

A group of people with early-stage Alzheimer's disease received recognition from the governor of Illinois for helping first graders develop their reading skills. Although these older adults experienced memory loss, they read to the children, listened to the children read, and provided assistance with words that the children did not know. Both the leaders of the group and the school recognized the potential of people with dementia to contribute and make a difference in the lives of the children.

It is too often assumed that people with dementia are unaware of what is going on around them. People with Alzheimer's disease have expressed concern or pleasure about a story that they saw or heard on the news or some event in their family life. In a discussion with people in an early-stage Alzheimer's disease group, a neurologist was surprised that the group members were most interested in research projects that focused on causative factors for generativity reasons. One woman expressed the concerns of the group when she asked, "Is there anything that we can do to help our children and grandchildren avoid getting this disease?" To help people maintain a sense of connectedness and address the need for fulfillment, it is important that caregivers, professionals, and family members facilitate opportunities to make contributions.

## RECREATING OR RENEWING A PHILOSOPHY OF CARE

The above examples of people's concerns about making a contribution to others directs attention to the consideration of all of the human needs that Maslow identified.

Focusing on love and belonging, self-esteem and fulfillment, and physiological and safety needs, we can begin to evaluate whether the organization's philosophy of care needs to be revised or whether we need to renew our emphasis on it.

Creating or recreating a philosophy of care should involve not only the organization's leadership but everyone who is a part of the organization, including staff and people who are receiving care and affected by the organization (e.g., families, volunteers, regular visitors). Only by casting a broad net can we explore and consider all of the values that are important to people connected to the organization. This diversity of input helps the organization's leadership to create a philosophy of care that is real and can become a cultural reality for everyone in the organization.

## MOVING A PHILOSOPHY OF CARE
## FROM PAPER TO CULTURAL REALITY

To develop and live a philosophy of care to the point at which every staff member internalizes it is a lengthy and sometimes challenging process. It is, however, a truly important process and well worth the ongoing work that is necessary to ensure that it becomes a value system that is shared by everyone. Moving philosophy from a document to a way of life in an organization may require a fair amount of cultural change. Change is almost always difficult and somewhat stressful. Therefore, we need to appreciate the dynamics of change and develop ways to gain acceptance of doing things differently. The difficulty in implementing change should not be under-

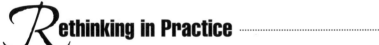

### *R*ethinking in Practice

*Creating opportunities for contributions to the community*

*The contributions that people with dementia can make to organizations in the community create a list far too long to be described here. All kinds of organizations in all communities need and welcome volunteer assistance. The kinds of volunteer assistance that can be provided depend on the retained skills of the people with dementia and the willingness of the staff to see them as people with something to contribute rather than as people with needs to be met.*

Call community organizations and ask what kind of help is needed.
Identify which people have the retained skills that are needed to do a task identified as a need by a community group.
Invite people with the necessary retained skills for the task to help with the project.
Organize the task in a way that provides a successful experience for everyone; break the task into manageable parts that fit the retained skills of group members.
Arrange the location of the work to best suit the abilities of the people in the group. Some people may be able to go to the community site, and others may be able to contribute most comfortably from the program site.
Publicly recognize the contributions made to the community group.

estimated and is not unique to those who care for people with dementia. Numerous volumes have been written on the topic of organizational change. A visit to an Internet bookseller unearthed 1337 books with "organizational change" in the title.

In general, change is most likely to be accepted if people who will be implementing the change are involved in the decision making and believe that the change fits their situation. It also is important to recognize and acknowledge the downside of and barriers to change and understand that problems will occur. Although implementing a philosophy of care that incorporates the beliefs and values advocated has many benefits for both people with dementia and those who care for them, it is not a utopian solution. Critical in any successful change process is that there is clear and continuous communication among everyone involved, especially as problems occur.

When the goal of having staff share common values about providing care is attained, it must be protected or it can easily slip away. Living a vision or philosophy of care is a process that requires passion and must be "lived convincingly, not just proclaimed" (Peters, 1987). As more attention is paid to the philosophy of care, the values in it will become an integral part of everything that the organization does clinically and administratively. For example, the organization's continuous quality improvement program will be based on the values described in the philosophy of care.

An emphasis on outcomes by leaders in an organization is yet another way to emphasize the importance of living a philosophy of care. The focus of our philosophy of care is the person with dementia; therefore, it naturally follows that the

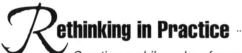

# ethinking in Practice

## Creating a philosophy of care

*The values that form the basis of a philosophy of care are both person centered and group centered. The development of a philosophy of care is an untidy, creative process that may seem at times more diffuse and chaotic than focused and businesslike. However, if one sticks with the process, points of convergence occur and ways to implement the philosophy into everyday life become clear.*

*Get everyone involved and find out what is important and valued by everyone who can be invited to help. Ask questions about what people want and do not want, what they like and do not like about experiences with this organization, and others. Watch people's responses to care, pay attention to verbal and nonverbal communication, and gather information from every available source.*

*After obtaining all possible input, begin the process of condensing and clarifying the information, continuing the process until the essence of all that has been expressed is clear. At this point a philosophy that can truly be lived will begin to take shape.*

*Ask staff to describe ways that the values in the philosophy can be demonstrated in day-to-day care provision. Explore the subtlety of the values expressed with staff, and examine which actions, behaviors, and attitudes are in accordance with the philosophy and which are not.*

focus of program evaluation also should be the person with dementia. Outcome measurements that focus on the person receiving care rather than on process measures, which focus on the person providing care, must be developed. Traditionally, the focus of evaluation was the care process, which called attention to the actions of the person providing care. However, research funded by the Agency for Health Care Policy and Research (1995) found few correlations between processes and outcomes of care.

Because outcome measurements are a relatively new form of program evaluation, it is tempting to rely on the familiar (e.g., conducting satisfaction surveys, measuring physiological responses to care). Although these measurements are certainly important, it also is critical that we develop ways to measure other equally important (or perhaps to the person with dementia, more important) responses such as the use of retained skills. The primary purpose of using outcome measures as an evaluation tool is to help focus attention on areas where improvement may be needed; therefore, measuring the use of retained skills will not only help evaluate the effectiveness of our programming but it also will emphasize its importance.

If attention is paid daily to the core values that have been determined to be essential in the provision of care, many of the problems that are all too frequently considered to be inevitable in dementia care will be avoided. As we relate to the person rather than to the disease, treating people with dignity and respect and muting control issues become a natural part of providing care. For instance, we know that Bernice feels comfortable and cared about when she walks in and announces, "I is home." If she gets tired after lunch, she finds a comfortable chair, puts her feet up, and takes a short nap. Her nap, which she takes instead of participating in an activity, is not negative or problematic, and it does not mean that staff are ignoring her. It means that her needs for rest and making her own decisions are respected.

In contrast, if Jim is doubled over in his wheelchair "sleeping" all day and staff accept this behavior because "he won't participate," we are not living by our philosophy. To live our philosophy, we must determine what retained skills Jim has and use our creativity to find activities that provide an opportunity for him to use those skills. As a culture of caring is established and everyone shares the same values, the way care is provided will be affected profoundly. We will not just go through the motions or make sure that care is provided in technically correct ways. The culture will be focused on caring for people we work with, and we will demonstrate this focus in big and small ways every day. We also will look beyond the disease and find ways to connect with and support the individual with dementia.

## REFERENCES

Agency for Health Care Policy and Research. (1995). *Characteristics of nursing homes that affect resident outcomes* (AHCPR 92-0008). Silver Spring, MD: Publications Clearinghouse.
Cohen, D., & Eisdorfer, C. (1986). *Loss of self.* New York: New American Library.
Davis, R. (1989). *My journey into Alzheimer's disease.* Wheaton, IL: Tyndale Press.

Dimnet, E. (1932). *What we live by* (p. 14). New York: Simon & Schuster.

Dunham, J., & Klafen, K. (1990). Transformational leadership and the nursing executive. *Journal of Nursing Administration, 20*(4), 28–31.

Freud, S. (1972). *A general introduction to psychoanalysis.* New York: Pocket Books.

Hammer, M., & Champy, J. (1993). *Reengineering the corporation.* New York: Harper Business.

Heiss, G. (1997). *Finding the way home.* Fort Bragg, CA: QED Press.

Jackson, P., & Delehanty, H. (1995). *Sacred hoops: Spiritual lessons of a hardwood warrior.* New York: Hyperion.

Kidder, T. (1993). *Old friends.* Boston: Houghton Mifflin.

Kitwood, T., & Benson, S. (1995). *The new culture of dementia care.* London: Hawker Publications.

Lubinski, R. (Ed.). (1991). *Dementia and communication.* Philadelphia: B.C. Decker.

Maslow, A. (1954). *Motivation and personality.* New York: Harper & Row.

Mitchell, P. (1977). *Concepts basic to nursing.* New York: McGraw-Hill.

Patient Self Determination Act of 1990, PL 101-508.

Peters, T. (1987). *Thriving on chaos: Handbook for a management revolution.* New York: Alfred A. Knopf.

Ryden, M.B. (1998, July/August). A theory of caring and dementia. *American Journal of Alzheimer's Disease*, 203–207.

# $\mathcal{R}$ ediscovering the Soul

*The mind tends to go off on its own so that it seems to have no relevance to the physical world. At the same time, materialistic life can be so absorbing that we get caught in it and forget about spirituality. What we need is soul, in the middle, holding together mind and body, ideas and life, spirituality and the world.*

*Marsilio Ficino[1]*

Many people are interested in exploring their inner selves and enhancing deep, soulful experiences. For some individuals, it is an ongoing challenge to experience intimate encounters. However, for many people with Alzheimer's disease and their caregivers, it is the opposite experience. Deeper or soulful feelings, experiences, and interactions are part of their everyday lives, although they may not realize that they are at the time. Amid the many losses that often become the focus of their lives lie miraculous gifts—a pathway to the soul and an accelerated opportunity for deeper thought and connection. Growth and development await people who are facing Alzheimer's disease. To achieve this growth, however, we must learn to recognize soulful experiences, support their existence, and connect with them.

## DEFINING THE SOUL

It makes sense to begin with the soul and how it relates to our lives. The soul can be thought of as a place inside each of us where deeper thoughts and feelings exist. It is a place where we go to think, feel, and communicate on a different, more intimate level than our everyday existence. It is a place that encourages us to free our minds, feel with our hearts, and experience the moment, recognizing the extraordinary in the ordinary.

---

[1]As quoted by Moore, 1992.

The soul has individual, social, and cosmic dimensions. It can be a state, quality, perspective, or view (Moore, 1992). It is a place where we go to question and search and experience a slower-than-usual pace, harmony, and wholeness. In addition, it is the part of us that keeps us balanced and tempers our egos with a sense of humility.

The soul is a part of us that is rich with life and love. It is the essence of our self, our center, our core being—who and what we really are. It is our most vulnerable place, where we trust ourselves and others. The soul is the place in which the highest level of personal growth and development occurs. When this inner growth takes place, it leads to external action, action that comes from soulful reflection.

Many people believe that the soul is synonymous with religion. Although the soul refers to a spiritual entity, it is not the same as religion. Religion can be described as an organized method of practice, participation, and structure that defines and facilitates what we believe (Seicol, 1995). Spirituality is an internal sense of identity that is awakened through our interactions with ourselves, others, and our God—a self-discovery. The soul is spiritual in nature because it is the part of us that feels, experiences, and communicates on our deepest and most intimate level.

Throughout our daily lives, we can easily become preoccupied with such details as work, money, or repairs and often overlook the soulful aspects. Technology continues to take us further away from our self and our basic way of living. We may become blind to opportunities to experience powerful encounters because of our constant pursuit of a destination or end product that we think is needed or desired. We may grow unfamiliar with our deepest self and our purpose and no longer acknowledge or experience this basic, authentic, and loving way of life.

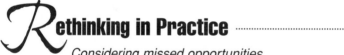

# *R*ethinking in Practice

### *Considering missed opportunities*

*In our lives and caregiving situations it is easy to become preoccupied with minor concerns and miss the simple yet significant possibilities of deeper, more meaningful thoughts and experiences. We can become so focused on one thing that we lose sight of or miss out on other possibilities. Consider the following scenarios and others like them:*

Recall how many times you have been on your way home from work and allowed yourself to become frustrated with heavy traffic; meanwhile, a beautiful sunset was coloring the sky beside you.

Think about a time when you became frustrated with a person for not doing something exactly the way you wanted, when it really did not matter how it was done.

Reflect on a situation when you shied away from interacting with a new person because he or she reminded you of someone else, but when you finally met the person, he or she was totally different from what you expected.

Explore a time when you had a disagreement with a friend or relative and held a grudge, and you missed out on significant events in each other's life.

Think about a time when someone with dementia was sharing something intimate with you, but you were too busy to listen or preoccupied by thinking about your next task.

## EXPERIENCING THE SOUL

The soul is deep but attention to it is simple (Moore, 1996). Everyday events can deepen into experiences of the soul. These experiences come in many forms and look different to different people. In general, an experience of the soul occurs when you become immersed in a thought, feeling, or experience and lose awareness of yourself. Nothing else seems to exist except that moment—time stops. You are completely enveloped by the moment, captured in an eternal present.

To experience the soul, clear your mind and become totally involved in the reality and ecstasy of the moment. Submerge yourself in the present, and allow yourself to breathe and feel the same air and emotions as though you are one with the moment. By doing this, you become centered and present with a deliberate attentiveness and embrace the moment with an open heart and a beginner's mind (Jackson & Delehanty, 1995). At the same time, you allow the questions within you to surface but do not become preoccupied with their meaning. From the perspective of the soul, finding meaning is less important than experiencing meaningfulness, and searching is more important than knowing (Suzuki, 1970). You learn to recognize and celebrate the unique and miraculous in everyday events, and allow imagination and reality to become one entity. You lose yourself and, at the same time, find your self.

The situations described in the exercise below are a few of the many possible paths to deeper experience. They are examples of common soulful experiences or ways of bringing the soul to life. These instances seem rare, but they do not need to be; we have access to them every day. It is important to be open to these experiences, provide space in our lives for them to take place, and allow them to influence our actions and interactions.

## ACTING FROM THE SOUL

Once you experience the soul, you may find yourself communicating from this feeling. Communicating from the soul involves transferring deeper thoughts, feelings,

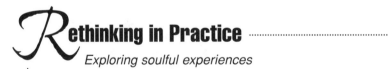

*Exploring soulful experiences*

*Paths to the soul are diverse and filled with opportunities for growth, development, and new experiences. They are illustrations of true connections with people, places, and things. We can tap into these opportunities in many ways. Consider some of the following avenues and others like them:*

Being awed by the sun setting over the ocean or by waves crashing against rocks
Losing track of time when walking along the beach, gazing at stars, or reading a book
Becoming so intrigued by a piece of art or music that you felt that you were part of it
Meeting someone for the first time and feeling entranced by his or her every word
Finding comfort in or being drawn to a person as you listen to him or her share thoughts and experiences with you

and experiences into action and interaction. It is allowing your thoughts and feelings to influence your behavior. Acting from the soul occurs with or without intention, consciously, or naturally in response to thoughts and experiences. At times, a feeling of the soul is acknowledged first and then acted on, or it may be an immediate reaction to a soulful experience. In either case the true voice of the soul is reflected in action, and its home is seated in the heart.

Connecting with the soul is a difficult concept to describe, but you know when it happens. Once you begin to communicate from the soul, you feel a connection that compels you to action. These are times when your soul, or inner world, clearly connects with the external world, when you connect center to center and heart to heart with another person or thing. Keep in mind that if given the space, souls always will be responsive to one another because they come from the same soul (Moore, 1996).

The ongoing challenge in our lives lies in continuing to live and act from the soul, which can be difficult when we allow petty grievances or differences to get in the way or when we become preoccupied with concerns and needs that are of little consequence. We must continually remind ourselves to look at things differently so that we will act differently. We must challenge ourselves to look at situations and experiences with a new set of eyes. These constant reminders can become an essential way of life when we are or someone we know is confronting Alzheimer's disease.

## NOURISHING THE SOUL

To experience the soul we must nourish it, much as one nourishes a plant with water and careful attention. Nourishing the soul means acknowledging our inner spirit,

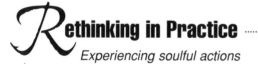

# $\mathcal{R}$ethinking in Practice

*Experiencing soulful actions*

*Acting from the soul usually begins with an experience or an action. Think about times you have acted based on an experience. Consider the following questions to help you to recognize times when you have acted from the soul. Read the following questions, then think about how you felt before, after, and during these experiences:*

Have you ever read a book, seen a movie, or heard a story that influenced the way that you behaved in the future?

Have you ever felt as if you knew exactly what someone was saying or needed, without him or her speaking a word?

Have you ever felt someone else's pain or emotion by watching him or her, talking with him or her, or listening to his or her journey?

Have you ever shared an experience of the soul with someone else and never discussed it, but knew that you both felt it?

Have you ever changed your approach to working with someone with Alzheimer's disease based on a situation or interaction with another person (or the same person)?

freeing the space around it, and giving it the opportunity to emerge, develop, and express itself. Simply put, we must enable ourselves to fully experience the moment by being open and allowing it to shape the way that we think and act. Our thoughts and actions are influenced by our experiences of the moment.

Nourishing the soul enables us to think, experience, and act in different ways, to move away from our everyday existence. For many people with Alzheimer's disease, being present in the moment is their usual way of being. Soulful encounters and experiences can be a natural part of the disease process for people with Alzheimer's disease and for their caregivers.

At first, experiencing and communicating with the soul may seem odd. Some people, especially people with Alzheimer's disease and their caregivers, may even find themselves struggling with the soul and trying to hold back powerful experiences because they feel strange or unusual. At certain points in the disease process, people with dementia and their caregivers may perceive soulful experiences and connections as weaknesses or disabilities. They may cover up the experiences, deny their existence, or become frustrated or upset when they occur. This can be the case, especially early in the disease process, when individuals and family members are trying to make sense of what is happening to the person with the disease and learning to cope with the many changes that are brought on by dementia. Both caregivers and people with Alzheimer's disease can grow more comfortable with these

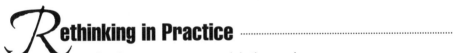

# $\mathcal{R}$ethinking in Practice

*Reflecting on ways to nourish the soul*

*There are many different ways to nourish the soul so that opportunities for soulful experiences can take place. Below are some suggestions to nourish the soul and allow soulful experiences to happen.*

Experience the moment. Become immersed in and fully open to the immediacy of an experience, and allow yourself to be present in the here-and-now. Welcome the uniqueness of the moment, and embrace the wonder of it.

Become less preoccupied with your mind. Allow yourself to feel from your heart. Let go of your ego.

Become quiet. Listen to the silence. Go inward to think, question, and search.

Recognize the inner beauty of other people and things. Look beyond the surface or exterior. Notice the extraordinary in the ordinary, the opportunity within the crisis. Celebrate the magnificence of existence.

Simplify things. Enjoy *being* rather than *doing*. Give up control and become flexible. Become vulnerable and trusting.

Be expressive, creative, and emotional. Experience things freely. Allow yourself to see the humor in a situation and take things lightly.

Love unconditionally, and become willing to express your emotions.

Sit quietly with an inspirational text or prayer book. Meditate.

Accept, relate to, and connect with others. Forgive and be compassionate.

experiences and not resist them as much. Embracing the possibilities of the soul is not always an easy or welcomed transition; it means letting go of how we think we are supposed to be or act and celebrating the moment and savoring the connection.

Some Alzheimer's care guidebooks, including this one, essentially encourage us to assume the qualities of the people with the disease; to learn from the way they must live their lives because of Alzheimer's disease. These books advise us to be creative and flexible and to make adaptations in our interactions. In a sense they tell us to trust ourselves to be authentic; they encourage us to experience our soul. We need to start thinking that Alzheimer's disease also can give to people, not just take away. It can open powerful new possibilities of relating to others in ways seldom experienced before onset of the disease.

## CONNECTING ALZHEIMER'S DISEASE AND THE SOUL

Many people with Alzheimer's disease experience soulfulness and communicate from the soul. The disease process eventually forces them to live this way. They may retreat from an intellectually based existence to a place of inner riches and spiritual freedom.

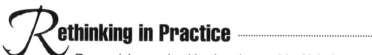

## *R*ethinking in Practice

*Recognizing and cultivating the soul in Alzheimer's care*

*Alzheimer's disease can offer a person many soulful experiences and connections. Think about instances when your interactions with someone with Alzheimer's disease, a family member, or even a fellow caregiver seemed somewhat different, yet more significant or powerful. At these times we can acknowledge the soul, either deliberately or by chance. To begin to look at Alzheimer's care differently, reflect on and discuss the following examples. Think about ways to support these types of experiences and make them possible in daily care.*

When you felt totally connected with a person with Alzheimer's disease, and when you saw that connection in the person's eyes or face or even felt it in your heart

When you knew a person's need without him or her saying a word, or when you knew how to respond without having interacted before

When you were lost in the moment while interacting with someone with Alzheimer's disease or a family member

When you allowed yourself to simply be with someone with Alzheimer's disease and to focus on what he or she found important or meaningful

When you felt the power and soul of touch

When you felt someone else's pain, embarrassment, or frustration

When a person with Alzheimer's disease was able to sense that something was bothering you, whereas friends and colleagues did not notice

When you were part of a "magical moment" but could not describe it or felt funny describing it to others

When you saw two people with Alzheimer's disease relating to each other in a different or special way

In a sense they can experience a reawakening or a returning to a more genuine and authentic existence. They can connect on both a deeper and simpler level—heart to heart or soul to soul, rather than mind to mind. Those who care for people with Alzheimer's disease have the same ability to connect but may not realize it. Caregivers become preoccupied with the frustrations of loss and focus on what the person no longer can do; too often they overlook these powerful yet subtle connections.

The person with Alzheimer's disease has no other choice than to live in the moment. At times, past and future lose their significance, and the here-and-now means everything. This allows people with Alzheimer's disease to take part in the ultimate existential experience—to be totally present in the moment. On other occasions, the uncommon blending of the past, present, and future shapes the here-and-now. Therefore, the way most of us live, with a linear chronology of time and distinct compartmentalized segments of past, present, and future, needs to be altered. This way of existence is an ongoing challenge for caregivers as they try to alter habitual ways of thinking and acting and become more open, flexible, and responsive to fleeting, ever-changing moments and events. If the moment means nothing later, in a sense it means everything now. The key is to allow the moment to happen, share it, and remain open to the possibilities.

The person with Alzheimer's disease needs life to be simplified. He or she may enjoy *being with* someone rather than constantly *doing* something. The product is no longer as important as the process; presence means everything. This concept is a challenge when people interact with a person with Alzheimer's disease, particularly when they try to make the person complete tasks, insisting on a tangible product, or to participate in a logical and purposeful conversation.

People with Alzheimer's disease also are able to let go of the ego and accept, relate to, and connect with other people more authentically. Often, other individuals are perceived without titles, labels, or skin color; they are simply other individuals. Many times their inner beauty is recognized and appreciated, and people accept one another unconditionally. Many of us struggle throughout our lives to live free of prejudice and stereotyping and to allow ourselves to be open to and feel compassion for people who seem different. For example, Stan, a Polish American, and Celia, an African American, were in an Alzheimer's group. Their diseases were well advanced, and they were known to hold strong opinions of others who were different from them. Celia began to scratch her head and accidentally pulled off her wig. Stan noticed what she had done and walked over to her, took off his baseball cap, and placed it on her head. He then picked up her wig, put it on his head, and sat quietly beside her.

Alzheimer's disease is also a catalyst for expressiveness, creativity, and emotional freedom. People with Alzheimer's disease can be very passionate about their beliefs and concerns, and their passion can be misinterpreted as violence or anger. They also can appreciate humor as they are able to take life and, at times, their mishaps lightly. Grudges do not persist because the issues tend to disappear along with the moment. This can be a good example for many of us when we take life too seriously and are not encouraged to express our emotions openly.

Instead of trying to teach people with Alzheimer's disease to come back to our chaotic and often preoccupied existence, we need to allow ourselves to learn from them. Everything that they experience is not bad. We must join them in their world, model their behavior and interactions, and allow them to teach us how to live more simply again.

There is more to Alzheimer's disease than loss and decline, but, in general, we do not hear about it. What we do not hear is that the progression of loss and deterioration also is an evolution of growth and development; it is an evolution that many people never have the opportunity to experience because they deny it to themselves and to the person with the disease. Instead of looking at what is being taken away from us, we must begin to look at what is being given: more time, more opportunity for soulful thoughts, experiences, and connections, what many people struggle to achieve throughout their lives. What we must do is recognize these soulful times and be present in them. In short, the opportunity for caregivers to nourish their soul is reinforced daily by the person with the disease, who is the essence of a soul on its journey.

## LIVING FROM THE SOUL

As we begin to change the way we think, feel, and act, we make the experience of Alzheimer's disease better not only for ourselves but also for the person with the dis-

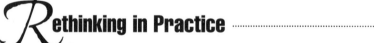

## *R*ethinking in Practice

*Embracing opportunities for soulful growth through Alzheimer's care*

*The soul is alive in Alzheimer's disease and available to us in daily care, however, we may not recognize it when we are focused on loss and decline and thus approach care in a closed and inflexible way. Think about ways to remain open to the following "soulful symptoms" of Alzheimer's disease and learn from people with the disease. Talk with your colleagues about ways to welcome and allow for these characteristics in daily interactions, experiences, and care.*

Living in the moment
Feeling comfortable *being*
Accepting opportunities and differences
Being creative
Expressing emotions freely
Embracing spontaneity
Welcoming simplicity
Loving unconditionally
Being curious and explorative
Letting go and moving on

ease. Our acceptance and recognition of a soulful dimension supports the person with the disease to embrace the journey instead of being forced to resist it. Most significant, we can view the person with Alzheimer's disease as more than a person with a cognitive impairment, but rather as our fellow sojourner, the person with whom we share life's journey. We can cherish the gift available to both of us: the unconditional willingness of the person with Alzheimer's disease to share with us fully, and in that sharing, teach us how to truly experience life.

We can learn to increase our own soulful opportunities and change the way that we approach life, which will affect how we relate to the people around us. As we continue to acknowledge the soul, our kindness, compassion, and new way of understanding and experiencing will encompass other aspects of our life and will affect those with whom we come in contact. We can learn to be more humane, compassionate, and respectful of others.

From a larger perspective, our thoughts and actions can begin to change the way others view people with Alzheimer's and other similar diseases. Our approach to the disease experience can serve as an example to others. As we grow and develop in our understanding, others will learn from our actions. Our behavior can serve as a model for others experiencing similar crisis-like situations, enabling them to emerge from them stronger and feel a sense of triumph. Even more broadly, as a society we can begin to destigmatize diseases that, traditionally, limit growth and restrict our access to it.

In time we may find new meaning in impairment and disease. Human suffering can be viewed differently. We can begin to see beyond physical and mental disability to recognize the unique individual and opportunity within every situation and encounter. In addition, we can view care connections differently, recognizing that they can nourish rather than exhaust and lead to growth, not burnout. We can then rejoice that we are beginning to live at the level of the soul, following its path, and allowing ourselves and others to be part of its incredible journey.

## REFERENCES

Jackson, P., & Delehanty, H. (1995). *Sacred hoops: Spiritual lessons of a hardwood warrior.* New York: Hyperion.

Moore, T. (1992). *Care of the soul: A guide for cultivating depth and sacredness in everyday life.* New York: HarperCollins.

Moore, T. (1996). *The education of the heart.* New York: HarperCollins.

Seicol, S. (1995, July). *Creating spiritual connectedness for persons with dementia. The changing face of Alzheimer care.* Presented at the 4th National Alzheimer's Disease Education Conference, Chicago.

Suzuki, S. (1970). *Zen mind, beginner's mind.* New York: Weatherhill.

# $\mathcal{R}$efining Care Approaches and Interactions

*It's important to know what disease the person has, but it's more important to know what person the disease has.*

*Dr. William Osler*

As individuals, members of a team, and citizens of a society, we have many reasons to be hopeful about the advances in the care of people with Alzheimer's disease and related dementias. As the 1990s end, the decade declared by the U.S. Congress as the "Decade of the Brain," there has been a growing understanding of some of the complex mechanisms that are the foundation of normal brain functions and of changes in the brain due to various neuropathologies. During this decade, an understanding of ways to provide increasingly effective daily care for people with progressive and irreversible dementias also has grown. Many opportunities and resources are available to develop or refine our skills in providing care. This combination of expanding scientific knowledge and more effective ways of providing care has set the stage for us to embrace a new era in dementia care. The accomplishments in the field of dementia care in the 1990s have brought it from obscurity to one of the most exciting places to work in health care.

Before the advances of the 1990s, care of older people with a dementia was largely a hit-or-miss proposition. Imprecise terms such as *senile* and *organic brain syndrome* were common and widely used to describe a segment of the population that was virtually ignored and "written off" by the formal health care system. Many people who were diagnosed as "senile" were provided with custodial care, services that sustained physical existence but provided little else. A sense of therapeutic nihilism prevailed, an approach characterized by a lack of hope and a sense of futility, foreshadowing the dire and inevitable decline of the diagnosed person (Cohen, 1988; Mace, 1987). When these people were cared for at home or in institutions, their caregivers usually were left to their own devices. Family members and staff received little information or direction from health care professionals, other than to medicate individuals to manage their "difficult behaviors," which were thought to be inevitable.

In the 1990s and beyond, the landscape of dementia care is alive with interest and opportunity—research grants, numerous drug trials, evolving clinical programs, and an emerging constellation of services from the early stages through the end of life. Although the clinical advancements have been considerable, they do not adequately meet the needs of the older adults who have been diagnosed. Only a small fraction of what we have learned has been widely disseminated; or if disseminated, this knowledge has not been widely translated into practice. Staff in many settings have a repertoire of available techniques and interventions, but often these are applied ad hoc. Despite the growing availability of a number of effective strategies that may work with some individuals, the lack of a coherent and comprehensive framework of care is evident. Such a framework would facilitate making care choices more logical and the process more systematic. To those who are new in the field, staff responses may seem, at first, to be a rather random selection process. Staff should be able to describe why they have selected a particular care approach (i.e., what they expected to achieve in matching an approach to a specific person with dementia). On one level it seems that some staff are willing to put into practice an intervention that they read about or heard of at a conference, without really taking the time to think about the rationale behind particular approaches. It is this lack of articulating the reasons behind the selection of certain approaches above others that is of concern. Although there is some element of trial and error involved, the person providing care should be thoughtful in deciding which way of responding is most likely to be successful. The likelihood of success is based on some general principles of good dementia care, combined with the particular and unique characteristics of the person with whom staff are working.

In many respects we in the field of Alzheimer's care find ourselves in the circumstance described by Kuhn and Polanyi (as discussed by Benner [1984]), that "knowing that" (certain scientific facts) is quite different from "knowing how" (what care is indicated). These two kinds of knowledge are different from each other. Despite many advances in the basic sciences, especially in the pathophysiology of dementias, the many newly discovered facts may not offer direction about how care is to be provided. In illnesses other than dementia, the impact is narrower and circumscribed; the treatment strategies flow directly from the biological impairment. For example, in the case of diabetes or high blood pressure, care interventions involve adapting the diet and supplying insulin or an antihypertensive. In Alzheimer's disease there is a complex brain pathology that can account for at least some of the symptoms that are seen commonly in people with this diagnosis. Unlike other diseases, knowing the causes of Alzheimer's disease does not guide care as clearly and directly. Therefore, from this knowledge we "know that" (i.e., what the dementia brain pathology involves); however, that information does not translate to "knowing how" to provide care. Because there is no effective treatment for the biological and chemical changes, care involves anticipating need and responding to the person in the context of his or her day-to-day life. This question of "knowing how" to provide care requires us to select a framework for care that employs the general state of knowledge and that implements care based on the situation and the available resources.

Borrowing from the framework of several influential authors in the field of Alzheimer's care, a systematic approach to care is described that can translate previously addressed concepts into the daily challenges of providing care. The approaches that follow are not intended as an encyclopedic summary but rather as an organized way of looking at various clinical approaches. The types of approaches that are selected should be based on a particular philosophy of care and best fit the person with dementia. Essentially, the next step in the refinement of dementia care requires us to be proactive in planning and describing our approach to providing care. We have moved beyond the point of simply reacting to behaviors. We have the knowledge base and experience to develop an overall plan for providing care in a systematic manner, a plan for understanding behavior, anticipating and meeting needs, and supporting remaining abilities.

## GUIDING CARE THROUGH
## THE PRACTICAL FRAMEWORK OF PERSONHOOD

Kitwood (1998) honed a conceptual approach to care that provides staff with a way of thinking about the essential features of what they do, according to certain principles that guide care. Rather than randomly selecting from among various approaches, Kitwood describes ways that reinforce or support personhood and well being throughout the course of dementia. Instead of providing care in accordance with routines that are organized for staff convenience, efficiency, or some other staff-based criteria, he suggests that the focus should be on the person with dementia. He describes 10 principles that constitute a framework for designing and providing care. They are straightforward and clear and can serve as a guide for illuminating how everyday interactions, interventions, and programs can be enhanced.

Kitwood's framework provides a way for staff to focus not so much on what is done but on how it is done. It is almost as though the activities and commu-

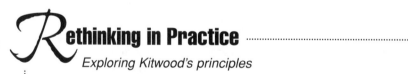

## $\mathcal{R}$ethinking in Practice
### Exploring Kitwood's principles

*In elucidating a framework for care, Kitwood provided an outline of ways to support personhood and well-being, noting the following activities: recognition, negotiation, collaboration, play, "timalation," celebration, relaxation, validation, holding, and facilitation.*

*It may be useful for staff to select several concepts for further discussion. Their selection could be based on areas where staff need some help in skill building, or staff could review and evaluate their overall compliance with the practices that support personhood. Staff also could evaluate whether their policies or accepted practices are designed for the convenience of staff or for the needs or preferences of those receiving care in the program. Discussion may point the way toward changes in policy or routines that are more responsive and person centered rather than to some other criteria for organizing care.*

nication strategies are vehicles that carry the real substance of care, the care of the person. The principles described by Kitwood assist care providers in critically evaluating how programs and communication strategies can be adopted and implemented to support the multidimensional person with dementia. These principles are in contrast to previous approaches to care that focused more narrowly on custodial tasks or symptom management. The Kitwood principles give us a language to shape individual clinical practice and the means to develop this capacity within an organized program of care. These approaches, along with a paraphrase of Kitwood's working definitions, are summarized in the paragraphs that follow.

## Recognition

Acknowledging the individual as unique includes using verbal and nonverbal responses, especially direct eye contact. It may be a simple greeting or it may involve careful listening over a period of time. Staff sensitivity is demonstrated when the form of acknowledgment is tailored to the unique persona of the individual and is consistent with that individual's capacity to receive and conduct a relationship with another person. The art and subtlety of acknowledgment should be reflected in staff's familiarity with that individual. Some people appreciate a respectful greeting using a title of honor that they cherish, such as "Dr. Jacobs"; another person may prefer a jaunty "Hi, Jack!" Staff should base these decisions on the recognition that seems to be the best fit for the individual. At a minimum, an acknowledgment should be made when care is being directly provided to the person. It also may be natural to do so if the individual passes by your office or passes you in the hall. For people who are easily overstimulated, less may be more beneficial, and you may develop a comfort level at which you share a gentle touch or a subtle wave.

## Negotiation

In the process of negotiation, the person with dementia is consulted about his or her preferences, desires, and needs. "Negotiation" should be a theme that is carried throughout everyday activities as well as individual situations. The key to negotiation is a process of openness regarding issues that, historically, may not have been a matter of choice for the person with dementia. For example, choice should not be limited to the more common and obvious selection of food or beverage but to broader questions of when a person eats and in what setting. Some negotiations may be problematic, such as those around issues over which staff typically have assumed control. For example, a situation developed in an adult day program that could have had dramatically different results if staff had not negotiated with George, as far as the limits of safety permitted.

> George held some paranoid views. One summer day, he refused to get off the bus when his group arrived at the day center. He seemed quite suspicious, and no amount of supportive encouragement could persuade him that he was

not in danger. Staff and even another participant approached him to offer food, beverages, a chance to use the bathroom, or to take him home.

After a series of unsuccessful efforts, a music therapist thought of the creative strategy of playing rock music, gradually increasing the volume at the back of the bus, where George had remained the sole passenger for 4 hours. This strategy was intended to resolve the situation in a way that did not diminish him. A staff member, who had not been involved in earlier efforts, walked by as the type and volume of the music began to frustrate George. The staff member offered to take him to a quieter place, and he eagerly accepted her offer. He allowed her to help him change clothes and welcomed her offer of food and drink. An hour after coming inside the day center, George was amiably engaged in a card game. Staff took him home several hours later, and there were no further untoward events that day. Staff felt justifiably proud. The situation was resolved by negotiation, in a continued effort to allow a solution to emerge that respected the choice of the person with dementia. Staff were able to keep their focus on the client's adamant desire to be in control, while balancing his need for safety and well-being. Most important, George finally was able to leave the vehicle on his own terms, instead of feeling controlled by others.

## Collaboration

The principle of collaboration requires making a conscious choice to work with the person in partnership. Care is not *done* to the person as if he or she were a passive recipient of care. Collaboration can include projects or personal care such as bathing. Sometimes a direct question or dialogue with the person is possible and sufficient in order to determine whether, how, and when the individual will be involved in some activity. The person providing care must gauge the comfort level of the individual by his or her response to the staff approach. The focus must include an appreciation of what the person with dementia wants or needs, apart from the staff's caregiving agenda. Staff must have the ability to monitor their own body language and how others perceive or respond to them. For true collaboration to occur, staff must be committed to the belief and value that the person for whom they are caring is entitled to be a partner in decisions involving his or her care, not merely a recipient or object of care.

Willie's family described him as independent, stubborn, and a loner. As his dementia worsened he became even more isolated, and increasingly, it became unsafe for him to be alone. He was very angry about being required by his physician and family to attend an adult day program. Initially, Willie resisted attending the program and expressed his opinion in colorful language and negative behavior. Because staff knew how Willie felt about this plan and what kind of person he was, they were able to approach him in a way that acknowledged and accepted him. Furthermore, staff let him know that they wanted to allow him as much control as possible. Willie often wanted time apart from the group. Sometimes he would sit alone on the patio and smoke a cigarette or sit at a table away from other members of the group. He would often observe and be attentive to conversation but at a distance that he chose. Staff always invited him to join groups but never forced the matter. Willie gradually warmed up to individual staff members and displayed a level of affection and sense of humor that surprised everyone. Because he occasionally inquired about a group member who was absent, it was clear that he felt connected and involved at some level. Willie became involved in group activities and outings more frequently, but he still needed space apart from others. He told staff he did not mind coming to the center but added with a wry smile, "I even like it some days; but don't tell my wife on me." When asked what made this change possible, he replied, "People seem to care about what I want, and they don't make me do things I don't want to do. I can tolerate people sometimes, but I need my privacy when I need it, and not when somebody else thinks it's okay."

## Play

Play involves spontaneity and self-expression for its own sake, with no particular goal other than its intrinsic value: joy in the moment. This interaction may be among the most difficult concepts for staff and families to appreciate and with which to feel comfortable. Many people who assist older adults with dementia find it imperative that they develop a capacity for sharing experiences that arise from happenstance and serendipity. For most adults, this capacity to enjoy simple events with abandon and unabashed glee can be a bit unnerving initially. The capacity to suspend logic often is a critical ingredient in living with dementia or in sharing enjoyable life experiences. It is possible to have fun in the moment, to create it, or to respond to situations lightly and share the humor as it presents itself.

In one special care program, the custom of the members of an exercise group was to say a prayer as a way of ending the group session and as a transition to lunch, which followed immediately. This prayer became an informal signal to the staff member who served lunch that the group meeting was ending and that it was time to invite the members into the dining area. One day, a member of the group wondered aloud whether the person serving lunch would know "to come and get us for lunch, if they didn't hear us praying." Another member of the group took the thought further by suggesting a prank: "Why don't we skip the prayer and turn the lights out and see what happens?" As the group became increasingly playful and mischievous, one member boldly suggested, "We could all pretend to be snoring if they do come in to check on us!" A few members thought that this might scare the person coming in. One person's comment was met with great laughter and full agreement: "They're a lot younger than we are; they can take it." A consensus quickly emerged. This idea was too delicious to pass up.

When the staff member who served lunch looked in on the group, she was genuinely surprised by the sight of a dark room with 22 people sitting in their chairs, eyes closed and snoring loudly. Then she heard muffled laughter and caught on to their game. Deciding to play along, she began to sing a lullaby. After just a few bars, the group members broke into fits of laughter. What had been a long-standing routine with clear expectations suddenly became an opportunity for a playful surprise. Both the planning and the results were a source of pleasure and warm delight for everyone involved.

## "Timalation"

Kitwood (1998) coined the term *timalation,* a hybrid of the Greek word *timao* (I honor) and stimulation. The emphasis in this approach is on using sensory modalities in interactions that provide contact, reassurance, and pleasure, when other forms of interaction are less available to the person because of advancing cognitive losses. Some people with a diminished capacity to express or understand verbal language because of dementia also may have sensory impairment (e.g., profound hearing loss, macular degeneration), which exacerbates the language problem. It is crucial that staff maintain communication through all of the other sensory channels that are available to help the person maintain his or her connection to others and to avoid premature and unnecessary decline due to understimulation and withdrawal from people and activities.

It is not clear which sensory channels may spark a response in someone with advanced dementia. However, knowing the person as an individual and introducing varying kinds and levels of stimulation often yield remarkable results. Sensory activities may be pleasurable and may facilitate a connection to a world that has been limited by the loss of verbal language and the cognitive and intellectual capacities for logical thought. The possibilities are limited only by imagination. We can explore ways to stimulate human emotion and connection through sight, hearing, touch, smell, and taste. We are challenged to find an avenue to reach inside someone or invite the person to come out of him- or herself. Contact can be elicited through a single sense; at other times we can combine several sensory inputs sequentially or simultaneously.

When staff use sensory stimulation it is important for them to eliminate or minimize competing sensory clutter in the environment to decrease distractions and to support connections through the use of appropriate sensory stimulation for each person with dementia. Sensory stimulation may involve helping an individual to savor a cookie or to luxuriate in having lotion applied to the hands or feet, accompanied by a gentle massage. An older adult with a love for flowers may respond to the fragrance of a fresh bouquet. Staff may offer to place it in the person's hands or brush a blossom against the person's cheek. At the same time, staff should try to allow time for the person to respond to and linger in the experience, if he or she seems to be connecting at that time.

## Celebration

The intent of celebration is to share planned or spontaneous events without concern for the artificial boundaries of the care-providing or care-receiving role. Using appropriate judgment, staff can share a part of themselves with the men and women with dementia whom they care for and care about. A pregnant staff member may share the progression of her pregnancy and shape and share the experience as though the members of her group were her friends. This vehicle may be useful for group discussions in that it provides an authentic way of eliciting wisdom and advice, sharing the joy of a new life, and sharing anticipation. The key is to be aware of whose needs are being met in the situation and ensure that the exchange is always in the interest of the people for whom we bear special responsibility.

## Relaxation

Differentiated by the lowest level of intensity and slowest pace, relaxation occurs when staff are involved and very much present with the person who has dementia. Nothing in particular has to be happening, but the feeling of welcome, accessibility, and comfort prevails. These interactions may occur during a lull in the schedule of more structured activities, at the beginning or end of scheduled personal care, and so forth. Relaxation may not involve conversation, but it always includes nonverbal communication that clearly conveys "we're together." This may be expressed in some form of touch or perhaps a playful smile, wink, or nod, which is sufficient to maintain or reinforce the sense of a shared and desired connection.

## Validation

Validation is a form of communication that involves exhibiting a high degree of empathy in a relationship with a person with dementia. It is an attempt to fully understand and accept the reality and power of the other person's frame of reference, even if the thought processes are chaotic or psychotic. This degree of active acceptance is one of the most critical skills for caregivers of people with dementia. Making an effort to "tune in" to what the person with dementia seems to be experiencing sets the stage for communication and activities. Validation requires us to appreciate who the person is and from that appreciation to select and modify our actions in accordance with what the individual seems to need most at a particular time. A person with dementia who is concerned and distressed about her "stolen" purse may be validated when a staff member spends a few minutes helping her look for it and then segueing the interaction into refocusing her attention over a bowl of ice cream. A caregiver should know how to validate someone but also know the proper timing for using it and how to make it appropriate for the individual.

## Holding

Holding essentially describes being with and for a person in distress. It is a message of affirmative support and addresses his or her unspoken fear of abandonment. It gives the individual a grounding and centeredness that may be lacking in periods of catastrophic upheaval, when feelings overwhelm the person. Holding is meant to encompass the literal meaning of physical contact but also must convey that the person with dementia is not alone, that you are there with or for him or her. The expertise found in this approach must be based on your knowledge of the individual. Sometimes a hug or an arm on a shoulder may be the source of distress or a possible means of alleviating the distress. In using this intervention we must be sensitive to feedback from the person we are trying to help. Our expression of support may be more or less physical, based on the individual's response to our efforts. If staff members try to convey support and comfort through touch and the person with dementia draws away, they must cease touching in favor of another, nontactile approach. Sometimes the mere presence of a staff member who has a warm, welcoming smile and a relaxed demeanor is more comforting to the person.

## Facilitation

Facilitation enables the individual with dementia to accomplish what he or she wants and needs to do but cannot do independently because the person is unable to initiate or complete the sequence of steps in the activity. The artistry of this approach is in subtly supporting or supplementing the person's effort to complete the task. Successful facilitation results in staff being satisfied in accomplishing what was intended, not in providing help.

Many excellent examples of facilitation can be found in the dementia care literature (Hellen, 1998). However, most examples concern cueing to support the accomplishment of self-care tasks such as eating or dressing or activities such as arts and crafts or active games. Facilitation also is required in interpersonal communication, although it has not often been described in the literature. Because much dementia care takes place in congregate settings, the ability to facilitate interpersonal communication is essential to help individuals retain their social persona. Thus, facilitation skills must bring together the knowledge of the person, a general understanding of the message that he or she is trying to communicate, and the capacity of other people to receive and understand this communication. This type of facilitation is more difficult to describe because of the rich texture of the context in which it occurs. One must be sensitive to nonverbal cues and the timing of when to speak, listen, and allow a productive silence.

The following example illustrates the power and beauty of successful facilitation.

A couple who were married for more than 55 years had a very loving and affectionate relationship. Ruth was feeling bad because her husband, Bud, who had Alzheimer's disease, could no longer tell her that he loved her. Bud seemed eager to proclaim his affection for his wife to others, but he could do so only in a very fragmented way that was unsatisfactory to him and confusing to the other clients in the group. He spoke occasionally in single words and sentence fragments when referring to her in an obviously loving way: "Beautiful . . . my girl . . . so good . . . a real peach."

On one occasion, Ruth came into the group as a sing-along was in progress. The staff asked her to join the small circle of singers. The staff member introduced Ruth to everyone, and Bud announced proudly, "I'm her husband!" With intentional timing, the staff member began to sing "Let Me Call You Sweetheart." It took a while for Bud to recognize the song and then, with dawning awareness, he seemed transported to another time. His eyes welled up with tears, and he stood in front of his wife for the duration of the song. He looked into her eyes and held her gaze and sang to her the words he could no longer say. For the moment, he was able to go beyond the language problems caused by the disease. The staff member knew Bud and understood his message and found a way for him to clearly express his love for his wife. At the end of the song, Bud was not the only one with tears in his eyes. In fact, the group spontaneously broke into applause, aware that they were both part of and witness to a very important moment.

## POSITIVE APPROACHES TO IMPLEMENTING THE FRAMEWORK

Taft, Fazio, Seman, and Stansell (1997) described seven domains or types of interventions that were identified by caregivers as the specific kinds of care they provide: social, psychological, functional, behavioral, environmental, medical, and cognitive. Although there were some differences in terminology, the interviews with caregivers revealed that there was considerable similarity of intent as well as specific approaches when compared with Kitwood's framework. This parallel was not drawn by Taft et al., but their findings matched Kitwood's framework of interventions that support personhood and well-being. The examples and discussions that follow are provided to help Taft et al.'s seven domains come alive.

In general, experienced staff in everyday practice do not consciously select from among these approaches. Often, it is difficult to elicit the precise reason that a staff member responds in a given way. Typically, approaches serve more than one purpose, and often they are woven into the fabric of daily care. In caring for people with dementia, you may find it useful to try to think about the reasons for selecting certain ways of responding to a given person in a particular situation and to evaluate the effectiveness and consequence of that response.

### Social Approaches

The interventions in the category of social approaches are defined as those that encourage interpersonal interaction and social functioning. In daily care these interventions include activities aimed at supporting purposeful engagement with people and projects, relating to a person in dynamic ways that help the individual stay connected with those in his or her environment, empathic caring, and supportive touch. In addition to "traditional" activity programs, there are ways to expand these approaches such as actively including participants in the orientation of new residents or group members and in discussions with students and visitors, in an effort to convey to them that this is "our place." Many people with dementia yearn to be of service to others. Depending on individual capacities, they can participate in assembling the adult day program's newsletter, selecting or arranging materials for the bulletin boards, and so forth.

## Psychological Approaches

Psychological interventions recognize and support the individuality and continued psychological functioning of the person who is living with dementia. Caregivers use psychological approaches when they are responsive to the person; view the world from the perspective of the person with dementia; offer choices, following the person's lead; and reframe or explain a situation to help a person cope better with it.

One of the most important changes in dementia care in the 1990s is a growing appreciation of the impact that Alzheimer's disease has on the person. There is a wide diversity in the human response to dementia. Many men and women are aware of their losses, and, like all human beings, they may express their feelings in words or behavior. One of our tasks as caregivers is to try to be open to hearing and receiving this information, providing people with dementia the opportunity to share their concerns in words and behavior, and providing the appropriate level of support. For example, when Florence was incontinent for the first time, she looked down at herself, initially denied that she was wet, and refused to accept help. Staff did not try to use logic or facts but simply accepted and supported Florence's responses. A few minutes into the episode, Florence broke into tears. She sat on the toilet, put her head in her hands, and wept. At one point, Florence, who rarely spoke clearly or coherently, said, very plainly, "I didn't know I was this bad." This is one of many examples of how people with dementia can have unexplained moments of coherence and insight. It is critical that we listen for these possibilities and be prepared to allow people with dementia the opportunity to express how they feel and to receive the support they need.

More and more often, John has felt confused, although he does experience some periods of lucid awareness. This juxtaposition in his mental state is perplexing for family members and staff. His caregivers are challenged in a special way to respond to the need to provide John with more oversight and assistance, while listening for and responding to the deeper levels of awareness and need that John may be experiencing. Once, after a particularly challenging weekend at home, John said, "I'm old, I'm tired, and I'm scared." These kinds of comments challenge us to think about how we can provide useful and meaningful psychological support for individuals.

## Functional Approaches

Functional approaches promote physical functioning or facilitate as much independence in activities of daily living as the person is capable of. Interventions include assisting directly or providing cues, supervision, or rest periods. Staff and family members need to experiment to find the best blend of assistance for the person with dementia. Often, subtle changes in staff approaches may elicit a different response.

If more than one person provides care, then it is important that they communicate with one another. This communication may expand or enrich the style of each caregiver and may lead to better care for the person, by offering the optimal assistance.

## Behavioral Approaches

Behavioral interventions are described as the nonpharmacological approaches that reinforce or promote desirable behaviors or alter undesirable behaviors. These approaches include caregiver responses such as diversion, noninterference monitoring, going along with the person, time away, delaying, confrontation, and using "therapeutic fibs." Taft and colleagues (1997) elicited and reported caregiver responses without commenting on or endorsing their merit. The authors noted, however, that confrontation rarely is a safe or effective behavioral approach.

This category of interventions is intended to avoid power struggles and confrontation. Behavioral approaches are predicated on the belief that prevention or early intervention is preferable to managing the situation once it has escalated. There are many subtleties to these approaches, for example, the artistry and impeccable timing of a caregiver's communication with a person with dementia. Nonverbal communication is an essential part of the success of these strategies.

## Environmental Approaches

Environmental interventions modify the physical environment to promote the safety and well-being of the person with Alzheimer's disease or a related dementia. Such approaches include modifying environmental stimuli, providing safety modifications, limiting access, providing personal identification, and using signage. The program design of one large adult day setting allows people with dementia to be cared for in discrete groups, or program clusters, based on their abilities, needs, and preferences. As an example, several groups at the center went on a field trip, and a few groups stayed behind. These groups, which usually are separate from one another, were condensed into a single group. Bette, a member of an Alzheimer's group, seemed decidedly uncomfortable. She fidgeted, was restless, and was overheard to say, "Oh, I don't belong here, with the real people."

On another occasion, there were a number of visitors touring a special care program. One program participant, usually quiet and calm, was uncharacteristically agitated. She said to no one in particular, "Why don't all those people go where they belong? They don't belong here." Being aware of the behavior and comments of men and women with dementia can communicate what level of stimuli is tolerable for people to function at their best in any environment.

## Medical Approaches

Medical approaches are defined as pharmacological interventions to modify behavior, improve cognitive functioning, or maintain comfort. In the climate of health care in the 1990s, concern was expressed that we try to look at behavioral approaches as a first level of intervention before considering medications. Anxiety and agitation in people with dementia has been reported in the literature for many years. Toward the end of the 1990s, however, more attention was being devoted to the presence of depression in older adults and to the growing number of diagnoses of coexisting depression in older people with dementia. Until we can establish benchmarks and a record of outcomes based on specific interventions, what proportion of decline in the health of people with dementia can be avoided or delayed long into the illness will remain unknown.

Long-practicing professionals believe that many behaviors that are attributed to dementia may be the result of medical problems that are avoidable and/or subject to remedy through more careful monitoring and management. These challenging behaviors can result from dehydration, undiagnosed infection (especially urinary infections and silent pneumonia), fluctuating blood sugar levels, and pain. Pain is a common human response to altered health and function. Older adults with dementia may lack the language or ability to recognize or identify the source of their discomfort. This pain may result from common musculoskeletal problems in aging, dental or podiatric difficulties, malignancies, and so forth. Staff should be alert to these potential health concerns, which require ongoing assessment, diagnosis, and treatment. Often, prevention or early recognition and intervention may eliminate or minimize discomfort. For example, a person with dementia with chronic arthritic pain could be placed on a routine schedule of pain medication. This might be considered because staff may not be able to see the symptoms of pain until the person has endured pain and discomfort for too long.

## Cognitive Approaches

Cognitive approaches are defined as those interventions that promote continued cognitive functioning, including reorienting and helping the person to remember. Although formal reality orientation programs have fallen out of favor, there are many opportunities to help people with dementia stay connected to the world. One way to do this is by focusing on facts and more generally noting landmarks—people, places, and events that the person seeks to clarify or is able to retain. The standard litmus test should be how the person responds to the facts and whether that person's needs are being met when we try to ensure orientation. In general, emotional reality is more important than temporal reality or facts.

## REFINING SKILLS AND DEVELOPING A PERSONAL STYLE

Our challenge is to articulate what the "gold standard" of care should be for people with dementia. We acknowledge in principle that there is uniqueness and individuality among those who share the same diagnosis; however, this understanding is not always described coherently and systematically. The framework of personhood may be broad enough to allow us to organize our approaches and give coherence to the kinds of care that are needed by people with dementia.

The term *refinement* is used to refer to the process of honing the art and skill of individual staff and the collective and coordinated expertise of staff as reflected in programs that care for people with dementia. Educational endeavors can only do so much to advance dementia care; the rest must be done by individual staff members who take on the responsibility to use the knowledge and tools and become skillful and proficient in their use. Each person must take these rough-hewn instruments (principles, guidelines, techniques, approaches) and develop his or her own style and technique in the practice of these instruments. There is no easy way, and no one right way, to provide care. Refinement involves internalizing the basics of care and allowing these seeds to grow within you as you develop your own persona, both as an individual and as a person who cares for older adults with dementia.

The actual provision of dementia care is a skill that comes only with practice. It is also an art, in the sense that there is an assumption that each individual will develop a way of uniquely expressing the principles of sound and effective dementia care. In Alzheimer's care practice and feedback are critical to develop excellence. We learn to refine our skills by practicing them, monitoring ourselves, and obtaining feedback from others who have achieved a level of competence. In this way, refining our dementia care skills involves a level of personal investment and willingness to seek out and employ input from others. This continuous self-awareness and mindfulness is essential to our personal and professional growth.

Presentations or general books about dementia must paint in broad strokes that the task of each individual staff member is to design his or her own palette of colors and select his or her own array of brushes. Only then is it possible, given some general rules of thumb, to select an intervention that is sensitive to the uniqueness of a given person and situation. It is imperative that you think through why one ap-

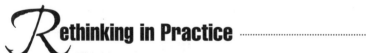

## $\mathcal{R}$ethinking in Practice

*Thinking about ways to refine skills and care*

*Because dementia care is always changing and is individualized, you must continually grow and develop, both in thought and action. Consider some of the following questions and others like them as you examine ways to refine how you provide care.*

What methods do you use to develop the skills necessary to perform your job?

After you attend a conference, watch a training video, and so forth, how do you employ the information you have learned? How does the information affect the way that you provide care?

What additional steps would be helpful to you to refine your dementia care skills further?

What do you do with newly learned information about dementia care to help make it your own?

proach may have advantages over another. Your knowledge is "portable"; in other words, you possess an ever-growing repertoire of possibilities. However, this knowledge is not particularly useful unless you also have knowledge of the person you are trying to assist.

Approaches to care are not effective if they are seen only as an ad hoc response to behavior. A person-centered approach to care acknowledges a multidimensional person, one who possesses a full range of human needs and capabilities and is able to contribute as well as receive assistance. Clearly, our care approaches must include a conscious intent and an overall design to provide authentic support for the health and well-being of the whole human being in the context of a shared community. These interventions must be selected and tailored to fit the person and the context of the situation. As relationships grow over time, it becomes clear that there is, or can be, enormous reciprocity in this kind of relationship. There is the potential for great comfort and satisfaction for people with dementia as well as for those who care for them.

Selecting approaches to care is an active and dynamic process that builds on a strong and complex foundation. This foundation must include a basic understanding of the pathophysiology of dementia and a philosophical orientation to care that results from thoughtful personal and organizational reflection about the underlying values that support all caregiving activities. This philosophy must express in practical terms the essential nature of the caregiving relationship. The foundation of care also must include the availability of textured and specific information about people with dementia in the full and rich context of each person's life. Each individual must be described and understood beyond the symptoms or stages of his or her dementing illness and basic profile of demographic data. He or she must be un-

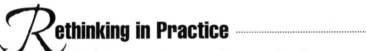

# $\mathcal{R}$ethinking in Practice

*Exploring ways to respond to care situations*

*Situation: A man with dementia starts to undo his zipper in one of your groups. How should you respond?*

There are usually a number of questions to be asked that would help pinpoint the likely causes of the problem and the nature of the individual and the setting or situation. All of these factors would influence the type of response. What other questions should be asked to assess what intervention would be the most appropriate in this situation? (For example: Is he newly admitted to the program? Does he have a urinary infection? Who are the other group members? How aware is he of his needs and his environment?) How would the answers to the questions influence a staff member's response? Would a standard procedure work for any person who showed this behavior? If not, why?

Discuss all of the possible ways that staff might handle this kind of situation.
Describe the reasons why a staff member should consider different ways to respond to the same kind of behavior.

derstood as a unique person who also is a member of a family and of many kinds of communities. Approaches to care must then be fashioned on this foundation and within a framework that guides care in a coherent manner.

## REFERENCES

Benner, P. (1984). *From novice to expert: Excellence and power in clinical nursing practice.* Reading, MA: Addison-Wesley.

Cohen, E.S. (1988). The elderly mystique: Constraints on the autonomy of elderly adults with disabilities. *Gerontologist, 28*(Suppl.), 24–31.

Hellen, C. (1998). *Alzheimer's disease: Activity-focused care* (2nd ed.). Boston: Butterworth-Heinemann.

Kitwood, T. (1998). Toward a theory of dementia care: Ethics and interaction. *Journal of Clinical Ethics, 9*(1), 23–34.

Mace, N.L. (1987). Characteristics of persons with dementia. *Losing a million minds: Confronting the tragedy of Alzheimer's disease and other dementias.* (U.S. Government Office of Technology Assessment, OTA-BA-323, 59-83.) Washington, DC: U.S. Government Printing Office.

Taft, L.B., Fazio, S., Seman, D., & Stansell, J. (1997). A psychosocial model of dementia care: Theoretical and empirical support. *Archives of Psychiatric Nursing, 11*(1), 13–20.

# $\mathcal{R}$econsidering the Meaning of Home

*Our true home is in the present moment. To live in the present moment is a miracle. The miracle is not to walk on water. The miracle is to walk on the green Earth in the present moment, to appreciate the peace and beauty that are available now. Peace is all around us—in the world and in nature—and within us—in our bodies and our spirits. Once we learn to touch this peace, we will be healed and transformed. It is not a matter of faith; it is a matter of practice.*

*Thich Nhat Hanh*

Good-quality dementia care consists of careful attention to many elements, one of which is the physical surroundings. Care providers are encouraged to create and families are told to look for a "homelike" environment. Design experts specifically describe the ideal place and make recommendations for colors, textures, and fabrics. Often, a great deal of money is spent on decorative wall hangings, nostalgic memorabilia, soothing wallpaper, and beautiful oak chair rails, all in a valiant effort to simulate the ideal home. At first glance these environments are very pleasing and often look like a home, especially to the potential customer. However, many people with dementia do not feel at home in these picture-perfect places, perhaps because the true essence of "home" is still not being conveyed.

What is "home"? What does it look like and how do we help foster it? For instance, when Bernice comes into the day center and states, "Yep, I is home," what does that mean to her, and why does she feel that way when she enters the center? Could it be that home is not a *place* but rather a *feeling*? If so, how do we explain the feeling of home, and how can we recreate and support that feeling for people with dementia in their care settings?

## DEFINING THE MEANING OF "HOME"

Home can be defined in many ways. A home is a person's principal place of residence, a private dwelling or habitat. It is the social unit formed by a family living together or the family environment to which one is emotionally attached. It is a familiar or suitable setting or a congenial environment. However home is defined, it consists of several components and a variety of meanings, all on a continuum. It is the presence of certain things and the absence of others. Also, home usually provides us with fundamental needs such as shelter, comfort, and nourishment. Ultimately, home is the place where our soul is welcomed, settled, and cared for. As one person with dementia said, "Home is not where you live but where they understand and care about you."

Several researchers have applied structure to the concept of home. Brawley (1997) described how home is not just a place but a concept of comfort and familiarity that nourishes body and soul and etches indelible memories in the mind. Dovey (1985) identified three themes of the phenomenon of home: order (how we orient ourselves in the world), identification (how we relate to our world in a meaningful way), and a dialectic process (dialectics between the inside and outside of home; dialectic is systematic reasoning that juxtaposes opposed or contradictory ideas, usually to resolve conflict). In other words, these themes of home include orientation, relation, and interaction, both inner and outer. These themes can provide a framework for home and help us organize it in a broad sense; however, an understanding of the various elements and components that make up home is essential to support and facilitate the feeling of home for people with Alzheimer's disease.

Home has been described as "the experience of a fluid and dynamic intimate relationship between the individual and the environment" (Carboni, 1990, p. 32). Carboni explained that the environment is made up of the physical, social, and psychological spaces around the individual. The relationships of the interactions and transactions between the spaces and the individual provide him or her with the critical connection to the meaning of life. Home can be discussed from a phenomenological perspective as a lived experience that possesses deep existential meaning for the individual. The relationship that makes up the experience of home emerges from the many interactions and transactions between the individual and the envi-

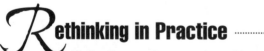

# Rethinking in Practice

*Reflecting on the meaning of home*

*Take a few minutes to think about the meaning of home. Ask yourself the following questions and others like them.*

What does home mean to you?
Which words would you use to describe home?
What are some of the characteristics of home?
Does the meaning of home change for you from time to time?
When do you feel most at home? What does that feel like? How do other people or your environment support or fail to support that feeling?
What do you get from home or at home that you do not receive in other places?
How do you continue to feel at home within the many changes in your life?

ronment and evokes different meanings for the individual. Home, then, can be described as the sum or totality of these experiences or meanings (Carboni, 1990).

The concept of home also can include the following meanings or experiences, each made up of different interactions and transactions (Carboni, 1990):

- *identity*, or the bonding of person and place
- *connectedness* with people, places, the past, and the future
- *journeying*, or a sense of reaching a destination
- *privacy*, or being in and out of contact with other people
- *power/autonomy*, such as personal freedom and decision making
- *safety/security* and predictability
- *lived space*, or the meaningful experience of space

These experiences can serve as a foundation to explore the concept of home and show us how it can mean different things to different people. We must take a closer look at the concept of being at home and examine the intricacies of this experience to better understand, support, and recreate it.

## BEING AT HOME

Being at home can be described as being in a familiar or congenial relationship or feeling relaxed, comfortable, and at ease (Zingmark, Norberg, & Sandman, 1995). A person is at home when he or she is in harmony with the surroundings, is acclimated to the environment, is on familiar ground, or feels a sense of escape or refuge from the outer world or community. Very simply, being at home has to do with feelings, relationships, and surroundings. As one woman with dementia said, "Home is where I can be myself."

A few authors (e.g., Zingmark, Norberg, & Sandman, 1993) have described the components of being at home, most significantly the relationships within these components. Together, these relationships help shape the experience of being at home. These components consist of meaningful relationships with oneself (e.g., inner self, calmness) and others (e.g., spouses, relatives, friends, pets). They also include relationships with time (e.g., day, period in history), objects (e.g., photographs, furniture), events (e.g., chores, work, hobbies, school), and places (e.g., house, neighborhood, town) (Zingmark et al., 1993). Meaningful relationships with each of the components allow a person to experience being at home; however, the level of significance or importance of each component varies from individual to individual. Meaningful relationships are a fundamental component of being at home and also affect the feeling of being at home. Of all of the previously mentioned relationships, those that pertain to oneself and others are significant and deserve special attention. Beginning with oneself, being at home can be a very internal feeling, where a person needs to feel and be at home with him- or herself before he or she can be at home with others or within a place. Others need to feel a family connection, family ties, and a clear identification of roles and responsibilities within that family. At times, feeling the presence of others is as meaningful or even more meaningful than the interaction itself, in other words, simply knowing that someone is there. Still others need to feel a connection with things that are known and familiar, which leads to many of the elements that allow us to feel at home (see next section). As an individual with dementia shared with the authors, "Home is where they know me."

## FEELING AT HOME

There are many elements of being at home that allow us to feel at home. As stated previously, feeling at home entails the presence of some elements and the absence of others. Alone and in combination, these elements help us to feel comfortable in our surroundings. A few authors have identified different elements of being at home (Zingmark et al., 1995). Recognizing and fostering these elements is fundamental as we support and facilitate the feeling of home for others, especially individuals with dementia. People must feel a sense of safety and security while having the freedom to make choices, take risks, and be themselves. They must feel in control and have the power and initiative to do as they wish. In addition, they must feel a sense of order, possession, privacy, and recognition. They need both physical and mental nourishment and rootedness and togetherness, or a sense of belonging and connection. Finally, they need to feel joy and harmony, knowing that things fit together and good times can and do exist.

Some of these elements and components may seem more like ideal attributes than reality. Home is not always a pleasant place or experience for everyone. At certain times, some individuals may have been part of a nontraditional or an un-

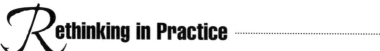

# *R*ethinking in Practice

*Supporting people with Alzheimer's disease in "being" at home*

*Home is more than simply a place; it is also a feeling. Many times, however, one must experience being at home in order to feel at home. Talk with your care team about ways that each of you encourage and support people with Alzheimer's disease in being at home. Consider the following components of being at home in your discussions, and share ways to continue to support and enhance meaningful relationships with these components.*

*What are some ways to support people with Alzheimer's disease in being at home by fostering meaningful relationships in the following areas?*

Oneself (e.g., privacy, being alone)
Others (e.g., social opportunities, group activities)
Time (e.g., deciding when to wake, bathe, or eat)
Objects (e.g., personal belongings)
Events (e.g., holidays, special times)
Place (e.g., creating own room, gardening, doing chores)

desirable home environment, which made their homelife unpleasant or atypical. The elements and components of home that they did experience may have been found elsewhere, such as outside the home (e.g., with friends or other relatives, at the library) or within themselves, making the feeling of being at home internal and individual. Therefore, comfort for them may lie more in others' respecting their need for emotional distance and space.

Being at home also has been referred to as *at-homeness* (Zingmark et al., 1993). At-homeness is when a person feels integrated or whole or that he or she has meaning, that is, when he or she feels completely at home. It is related to integrity, or sincerity and wholeness, and occurs when the many elements of home are in sync. This congruence can become stronger during different periods of our lives and depends on our experiences (Zingmark et al., 1993). At the same time, this feeling exists on a continuum, with homelessness on the opposite end of the spectrum.

## EXPERIENCING THE PHASES OF HOME

Throughout our lives, we experience different phases of home. Zingmark et al. (1995) identified four phases of home: being given a home, creating a home, sharing a home, and offering a home. At certain times the concept of home may have a

## *R*ethinking in Practice

*Cultivating the feeling of home for people with Alzheimer's disease*

*Many elements of being at home help us to feel at home. Take time to discuss ways that your care team and environment accommodates and supports the following areas or elements of being at home. It may be helpful to make two lists or columns—one for "place" and another for "feeling." Discuss each element in relation to each of the areas. For example, a locked outside door may address safety for home the place, but what about safety for home the feeling? What do you do to help people feel safe? Remember to think beyond the physical environment and consider the social and cultural aspects of being at home. Consider approaches, interactions, experiences, and the overall feeling of the environment. Continue to discuss some of the other elements identified by Zingmark et al. (1995) that are listed below:*

Safety (security, refuge, protection)
Order (arrangement, personal schedule)
Rootedness (grounded; belonging, ties)
Control (doing as you wish, influence)
Harmony (soothing, agreement, accord)
Possession (ownership, responsibility)
Joy (happiness, pleasure, delight)
Nourishment (meals, personal growth)

Privacy (keeping your own space, being alone)
Initiative (flexibility, spontaneity)
Togetherness (relationships, mutuality)
Power (control, authority, accomplishment)
Recognition (people, objects, smells)
Freedom (being yourself, making decisions)

different meaning. In addition, more importance may be placed on different phases as we experience or reexperience them. It is important to recognize the various phases of home and the significance that they may hold.

1.  **Being given a home:** The phase of being given a home is when a home is provided to someone. For instance, a child or teenager can be given a home by his or her parents. Also, someone can be given a home in a time of need or when he or she is ill. It is important for the person to feel welcomed and allowed to feel at home when a home is being given.

2.  **Creating a home:** The phase of creating a home is when a home is being created. It may be a continuous or evolutionary process because our lives are always changing. For instance, a child may create his or her own space within his or her parents' home or move out to create a home of his or her own. When a person marries, a home is created with his or her spouse. A person may model this newly created home after his or her childhood home, or, in some cases, it may be completely different. Also, with life changes such as illness or divorce, a new home may have to be created or a current home recreated. It seems important for people to be able to rely on home as life presents experiences.

3.  **Sharing a home:** The phase of sharing a home is when it becomes important to share a home with others. This phase can include starting a life with a spouse or partner; living with a roommate; having children; and/or taking in relatives, pets, or someone in need. The formation of a mutually reciprocal relationship is important during this time.

4.  **Offering a home:** This phase is offering a home to others. This phase can include inviting company over for parties or get-togethers, hosting holiday celebrations for families and friends, asking the grandchildren to stay over, or housing out-of-town guests. Being hospitable and making others feel comfortable and welcome is important during this phase.

These four phases provide structure to the overall experience of home throughout our lives. They demonstrate that people may have different needs or feelings of home at different points in life, depending on what is important to them at the time. In addition, the phases are fluid. This fluidity is important to keep in mind when interacting with people with Alzheimer's disease or a related dementia because each phase may have different qualities and meanings as the individuals experience or reexperience it.

## TRANSITIONING WITHIN HOME

Throughout our lives, we experience not only different phases of home but also transitions within home. For instance, we may move into a college dormitory, experience a job transfer, join the military, or marry. These life changes force us to immediately reexperience a different phase of home, with or without wanting to at the time. For people with Alzheimer's disease and their caregivers, these transitions can be even more significant because they are multiple, have a specific impact, and demand time for adjustment.

Think about the four phases of home in relation to the transitions that can occur during the course of Alzheimer's disease. People with dementia may be *given a home* when they need to move in with their adult child or children. They may experience *creating a home* when they move into an assisted living facility. They may experience *sharing a home* within a residential care setting. They may have to *offer a home* when, for example, a family member moves in with them. Therefore, for people with Alzheimer's disease and their caregivers, the phases of home can continually change, both internally and externally.

## EXPERIENCING HOME THROUGH THE PERSON WITH ALZHEIMER'S DISEASE

A person with Alzheimer's disease may mention home several times a day. In some instances the person may be looking for home or simply want to go home. This need becomes increasingly challenging when the person is already where he or she lives. The fact is that the person must not feel like he or she is at home. On some occasions, in looking for home a person may be asking for "mother." "Mother" and "home" seem to mean the same thing at certain times, that is, being secure, loved, and nurtured and feeling positive and safe (Brawley, 1997). In either case, the person is looking for something he or she does not have or feel at that moment.

## *R*ethinking in Practice

*Acknowledging the four phases and transitions of home in Alzheimer's care*

*Home can be organized into four phases: being given a home, creating a home, sharing a home, and offering a home (Zingmark et al., 1995). As individuals we experience these different phases in many variations throughout our lives, and the transitions that affect individuals with dementia can affect their feelings and experiences. Talk with other members of your care team about these phases and transitions of home and how they relate to the individuals for whom you care. Consider some of the following questions in your discussions:*

Have you ever thought about individuals being in different phases of home?

Do assessments, care plans, and programming reflect the different phases? How so?

What phases do individuals in your care environment experience the most?

How do programming and interactions allow for the different phases?

What are some ways that you can support individuals with Alzheimer's disease in these different phases of home?

What are some ways that care providers or other individuals with dementia can help others cope with transitions?

The experience of home for people with Alzheimer's disease has been organized into two categories. First, people with Alzheimer's disease may be *longing for home*, which can include memories of previous home/relationships, creating expectations of a future home, or looking for the present home. Second, people with Alzheimer's disease may be *on their way home*. This can occur when others leave for home, when they are feeling overwhelmed or abandoned, or when there is a lack of activity or interaction (Zingmark et al., 1993).

People with Alzheimer's disease also may experience homesickness or homelessness. Not feeling at home also has been referred to as homesickness (Carboni, 1990). Homesickness has been described as a defense against feelings of not being at home in the present. Many times this inner experience is directly related to, or caused by, experiences in the outside world. Homesickness is the direct opposite of being at home, or at-homeness. Homelessness is also the opposite of at-homeness, and lies at the other end of the continuum of feeling at home. Homelessness can be described as the negation of home, in which the relationship between the individual and his or her environment loses its intimacy and becomes damaged in some way. It evokes such meanings as nonpersonhood, disconnectedness, lack of journey, no boundaries, powerlessness or dependence, insecurity or uncertainty, and lack of personal space (Carboni, 1990). Many care environments unintentionally

## *R*ethinking in Practice

*Exploring care approaches for someone with Alzheimer's disease who is looking for home*

People with Alzheimer's disease commonly say, "I'm going home now." One reason may be that although where they live may look like a home, it may not feel like a home to them. Another reason is that their needs are not being met at that time or that an uncomfortable situation just occurred. Of course, the reason could be one of many.

Discuss with others ways to interact with people with Alzheimer's disease when they are looking for home. It may be helpful to think about a specific person with whom you are working. Ask yourself and others the following questions:

What else is going on (or not going on) when someone asks to go home?

Have you explored what home means to that person or what aspects of home he or she is looking for?

Does the person feel at home in that environment? Why or why not?

Is the person "longing for home" or "on the way home"? How would approaches or interactions differ in each situation?

If the person is longing for home, how can you recreate or share memories of what he or she is longing for?

If he or she is on the way home, what else is going on at the time? How can you help the person find home without leaving the environment (home the feeling versus home the place)?

create feelings of homelessness and homesickness via their approaches, interactions that take place in them, and surroundings (e.g., décor). Careful attention must be paid to the various aspects of being at home to identify how we can alleviate homelessness and homesickness while we encourage at-homeness.

Brawley (1997) suggests that we must begin with the "language" of home and change the way we speak about the environment. The language of home is quite different from that of a residential facility or health care environment. Words such as "corridors" should be called "hallways," as they are in the person's home of origin, and other rooms should have specific purposes (e.g., kitchen, living room, dining room). Settings should not be planned to reach for the ambiguous "homelike" but to try to achieve a humane and typical setting. Settings need to be designed for comfort, support, and healing of both body and spirit within a physically and emotionally safe place. With all of the changes taking place within the person with dementia and his or her world, it is especially important for him or her to maintain ties to the familiar and the comfortable (Brawley, 1997).

## UNDERSTANDING AND CREATING THE FEELING OF HOME FOR PEOPLE WITH ALZHEIMER'S DISEASE

Home is a complex phenomenon that can be described in many different ways, including themes, components, and phases. Each categorization further defines or organizes the overall concept more comprehensibly so that we can understand better what the experience is about. Understanding the concept of home can be challenging because each person's idea of home may be different and have a specific mean-

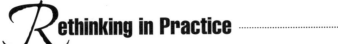

## *R*ethinking in Practice

*Creating a personal home within a care environment*

*The meaning of home differs from person to person. Home is not only a different place but also a different feeling. It consists of things like meaning, relationships, elements, phases, interactions, and experiences. It is complex but simple; a presence and an absence; the same yet different.*

*In our day-to-day caregiving, it is important that we allow for these differences, the uniqueness of home. This allowance can be challenging, however, when many different people are living in the same environment where the boundaries between public and private places become blurred and where leaving home and returning home are not always possible. As your care for people with Alzheimer's disease evolves and grows, challenge yourself and others to explore ways to support and nourish individuality within the commonalities. Hold ongoing discussions on how to allow for individuals' uniqueness within this sameness. Explore how approaches and environments can change, and explore ways to overcome potential barriers. Continue to supportively challenge one another and foster and celebrate the many personal homes within the broader home, your care environment.*

ing, especially during certain periods of his or her life. Some common elements are shared by all people, however. These elements help compose the universal feeling of being at home. This feeling of being at home is what we must strive to capture and recreate in Alzheimer's care. The key is to recognize the differences in the many applied meanings while we celebrate the similarities.

Time must be taken to find out what home means to each individual and to become intimate with what generates the feeling of home. Individuals should be given the opportunity to help create their own environments—physically, emotionally, and culturally. Families can help by sharing stories and their ideas of what home was like for the person with Alzheimer's disease. Staff must believe in, practice, and internalize this philosophy of care, and the facility's policies must reflect it and must be developed with enough flexibility for this to occur. In addition, various relationships with the different components should be explored and included in clients' or residents' care plans, such as accessibility to certain objects, interactions with certain people, or participation in specific events. Every effort should be made to identify what constitutes the feeling of home and to strive continually to support and recreate it. As eloquently put by a person with dementia, "Home is when I'm with people I care about and who care about me."

The feeling of home is internal; however, it is created or supported by many external forces, such as people, interactions, and physical surroundings. Home is much more than mere furnishings; it consists of relationships, interactions, and approaches. People must relate to one another in a way that supports the identified elements of home such as safety, togetherness, and harmony. These elements can be allowed for or supported by encouraging interactions, relationships, and environments that recognize and embrace these important elements. Care approaches must consist of the elements of home to help people with Alzheimer's disease feel comfortable and at ease or at home with their caregivers. All aspects of the environment—physical, social, and cultural—must be adapted continuously to honor these elements.

It is important to identify which phase of home the person with dementia is most closely associated with because significance may be placed on experiences during that phase. For example, if the person is asking for "mother," he or she may be more connected with the phase "being given a home" and may have different needs from someone who is tidying up and in touch with the "sharing a home" phase. Also, people may experience different phases on different days. Therefore, it is essential to identify the phase that the person is experiencing, allow him or her to experience it, and connect with him or her in that phase. Connecting with the person means supporting his or her experiences and relating in a way that fosters the many elements of home.

Connection, relationships, and interactions seem fundamental to every aspect of home that was examined in this chapter. Care providers must move beyond the physical environment when attempting to recreate home and must explore, understand, and support the emotional and cultural aspects of home. Only then can we begin to truly discover the *feeling* of home rather than the *place*.

# REFERENCES

Brawley, E.C. (1997). *Designing for Alzheimer's disease. Strategies for creating better care environments.* New York: John Wiley & Sons.

Carboni, J.T. (1990). Homelessness among the institutionalized elderly. *Journal of Gerontological Nursing, 16*(7), 32–37.

Dovey, K. (1985). Home and homelessness. In I. Altman & C.M. Werner (Eds.), *Home environments* (pp. 33–64). New York: Plenum.

Zingmark, K., Norberg, A., & Sandman, P. (1993, May/June). Experiences of at-homeness and homesickness in patients with Alzheimer's disease. *American Journal of Alzheimer's Care and Related Disorders and Research,* 10–16.

Zingmark, K., Norberg, A., & Sandman, P. (1995). The experiences of being at home throughout the life span: Investigation of persons aged from 2 to 102. *International Journal of Aging and Human Development, 41*(1), 47–62.

# chapter seven

# Reshaping the Environment

*The bird a nest*
*the spider a web*
*the human friendship*

*William Blake, "Proverbs from Hell"*

Environment is an important consideration when caring for people with dementia because symptoms such as memory loss necessitate providing a prosthetic environment (one that compensates for specific individual deficits) to support physical and psychosocial function. Much has been learned and written about how to design and create a physical space that can be therapeutic for people with Alzheimer's disease, including physical features that support retained skills and function (Brawley, 1997). Design principles for the physical environment have been clearly articulated and provide guidance in the development of physical space that helps mitigate loss in function (Calkins, 1988; Cohen & Weisman, 1991). Although the importance of the physical environment is recognized, it alone cannot compensate for the losses that are experienced by people with dementia or support their strengths to maximize functioning. Consideration must be given to the whole context of care, that is, the physical, social, and cultural environments and how they blend together to create a milieu that is supportive of the person with dementia. In *The Key Elements of Dementia Care* (Alzheimer's Association, 1997), emphasis is placed on the interplay of all of the components of the environment: physical (e.g., structural, finishes, flexible components such as activity supplies), human (e.g., staff, people with dementia), and cultural (e.g., activity programs; organizational policies, practices, and budget). It is the interplay of these components that determines one's experiences and feelings in any care setting. The goal is for all of the components of the environment to work together to maximize physical and psychosocial functioning and, more important, create the feeling of comfort and well-being that most people associate with home.

## RECOGNIZING THE IMPACT
## OF THE PHYSICAL ENVIRONMENT ON FUNCTION

The concept of the physical environment as being therapeutic is critical when compensating for a person's losses so that remaining skills can be used. In group care environments people with dementia sometimes are described as nonparticipatory, implying that the person chooses not to participate in a particular activity or task. Although this may be the case, these people also may not possess the capacity to overcome the environmental barriers and participate in the particular activity. For all care, including activities, to be effective for people with dementia, first, a supportive and comfortable environment that balances their internal and external realities must exist. Annie, a woman with Alzheimer's disease, told a staff member, "When you forget things, you worry a lot about doing something embarrassing . . . about what people will think of you." Concerns like Annie's are an all-too-common reason that people do not attempt tasks that are within their physical capacity. Feelings like these can be compounded or ameliorated by the environment.

It is important to recognize that environmental designs that are appropriate for some people with dementia can reduce function for others. Mazelike hallways,

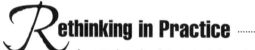

# *R*ethinking in Practice

### *Assessing the impact of the physical environment on function*

*When we accept the premise that a prosthetic environment is as essential to the functioning of a person with dementia as a limb prosthesis is to a person with an above-the-knee amputation, we begin to think about ways to use the physical environment as a therapeutic tool. Think about a familiar group care setting and discuss the following environmental issues:*

Describe ways that the environment compensates for cognitive, physical, and sensory losses.

Discuss some ways that the environment is a barrier to a person's ability to use his or her remaining skills.

Share ways to minimize environmental barriers that impair functioning.

*Because no single environment can be optimal for everyone, think about a specific person with dementia and ask yourself the following questions and others like them:*

Are wayfinding cues, such as signs, helpful for this person?

Does the place mat on the dining table provide space definition for this person or add confusing clutter?

Is the amount of ambient noise at lunch comforting or confusing for this person?

What information is needed to assess these kinds of environmental "fits"?

*There are many simple environmental modifications that can be made to maximize a person's functional ability. Considering the needs and abilities of a specific person, what modifications would help compensate for this person's losses and enable the individual to use his or her retained skills?*

designed as "wandering paths," can add to a person's distress, if directional signs and other wayfinding cues do not help him or her find the bathroom. This distress can often be detected in the person's tone of voice, or the person may be able to articulate the distress he or she is experiencing. One person with dementia, searching for the bathroom, said, "I want to do everything exactly right, but I can't find the right place." Such comments have led clinicians to believe that the inability to locate the bathroom may be a significant cause of incontinence. These beliefs were confirmed by research conducted at the Corinne Dolan Center, which found that people were eight times more likely to use a bathroom independently when the bathroom could be seen than when it was not easily visible (Namazi & Johnson, 1991).

A person who is easily overstimulated will not be able to function at his or her maximal capacity in a large space where multiple activities coincide with high levels of ambient noise. In fact, a person may be so overstimulated that he or she is hardly able to function at all. A person who needs a quiet environment to concentrate on a task will experience great difficulty eating meals in a large, noisy dining room. If those who are providing care to a person with dementia are not attuned to the impact of the environment on his or her function, they may easily and erroneously conclude that the person has a poor appetite or needs assistance in eating, when what is really needed is a quiet place to eat.

## RECOGNIZING THE IMPACT
## OF THE PHYSICAL ENVIRONMENT ON BEHAVIOR

Environment affects not only function but also behavior or actions. Socially and culturally acceptable behaviors and even the way we dress vary dramatically in different settings. We act and dress very differently in a church from the way we act and dress at a ballpark, a party, or home. The impact of environment on behavior is widely acknowledged in the fields of sociology and psychology, yet all too often its impact on a person with dementia is not considered as a contributing factor for a specific behavior or action.

The wife of a man with severe cognitive impairment described how he rose to the occasion at their daughter's wedding:

Holidays and special occasions had gotten to be very troublesome for him. The bustle of activity and the confusion inherent in large family gatherings sometimes seemed to overwhelm him, and he would sometimes act in unpredictable ways. We were very concerned about how he would respond at the wedding, but my daughter really wanted him to walk her down the aisle. Knowing the problems that could occur, we made a number of contingency plans (I would walk my daughter down the aisle if her father couldn't; the reception was held close to home so a friend could take my husband home if he got overstimulated, and so forth). I was very worried because he was really uncooperative before we left home; we even had a hard time getting him to put on his tuxedo. When we got to the church, everything changed. It seemed that he just couldn't comprehend that we were preparing for a wedding until we got to the church. When he saw the decorations and our daughter in her wedding dress, he announced, "I am the father of the bride!" Then he seemed to know what he needed to do. Not only did he walk his daughter down the aisle but he also stood in the reception line and told each guest that he was the father of the bride. He even danced with his daughter after dinner.

"Sundowning" and "catastrophic reactions" are terms sometimes used to describe symptoms that are thought to occur like the eruption of a volcano, without warning. When these behaviors are perceived in this way, little consideration is given to the environmental stimuli that may be a contributing or even a causative factor of the behavior. The perception of the behavior as a problem within the person, an inevitable part of the disease, rather than as a response to something in or lacking in the environment, greatly influences caregivers' responses to the behavior. If those who care for a person with dementia believe that the behavior is a response to an en-

# *R*ethinking in Practice

*Assessing the impact of environment on behavior*

Lucille was an active participant in an adult day program for older adults with dementia. Despite her memory loss, she was articulate and alert, and she functioned quite independently. A staff member from the center visited her when she was hospitalized with pneumonia. Lucille's primary nurse at the hospital had described her as actively hallucinating, requiring a psychiatric consult and medication. When the staff member spent time with Lucille, she found that environmental stimuli were contributing to the behavior that the nurse described. A bell-like sound could be heard in the hallway, and Lucille said that she knew the priest was coming with communion. She complained, "I can hear him, but they won't let me see him." Lucille thought that the bell-like sound was a bell being rung to announce the priest's arrival on the floor. The center staff member got Lucille out of bed, took her into the hallway, and showed her that the source of the sound was a floor-cleaning machine, not a bell being rung. Lucille's anger dissipated and she asked, "Well, why didn't someone tell me?" Although reasoning or reality therapy usually is not an effective approach for someone with Alzheimer's disease, it works in some cases, depending on the person's capacity. Because the adult day center staff member knew Lucille's capacity, she knew that it was an approach that would likely be effective.

Lucille's experience is not uncommon. People with dementia may be disturbed by something in the environment that they misperceive. It is our responsibility to help interpret or adapt the environment in a way that will decrease the potential for anxiety and distress.

Consider some elements in your environment that could be misperceived.

Consider some ways to help interpret these stimuli for specific people. How do these ways differ?

vironmental stimulus, then the person providing care accepts the responsibility to try to understand the distress or need being communicated by the behavior and to modify the environment, instead of treating the person or the symptom as the problem.

> During the holidays, Daisy became very distressed in the evenings and constantly tried to go outside "to get the children." None of the approaches that usually were effective with Daisy, such as reassurance or distraction, helped reduce her distress. Her anxiety would escalate throughout the evening and made getting her to go to bed a difficult task. Daisy's daughter was looking out the window with her one evening and realized that Daisy was focused on a set of lighted plastic Christmas carolers standing on the lawn. She asked staff to unplug the carolers. Within minutes, Daisy's distress dissipated. The behavior that had been described as sundowning by some actually seemed to be Daisy's mothering instinct to "take care of the little ones out in the snow."

## RECOGNIZING THE IMPACT OF THE SOCIAL ENVIRONMENT

What families and people with dementia want and expect from group care settings is that the client's or resident's basic needs are being met. In the authors' experience, one of the phrases that families most frequently use to describe a facility is "it was clean and didn't smell," which can be translated into a belief that their loved ones' physical needs are being met. They want their family member with dementia to be safe and feel safe. Beyond safety, families want social, intellectual, and emotional needs to be met. People with dementia want to be treated with dignity and respect, to have autonomy, to feel safe, to be able to help when they can, and to receive help when needed without feeling demeaned. None of the items described by families or people with dementia as being really important had anything to do with the facility's physical environment or design, other than cleanliness. In other words, a well-designed physical environment, although important, is not enough; people in the environment also must be responsive to the person with dementia.

It is the human environment, not the physical environment, that frequently has the greatest influence on the culture of a place and how people act and function in a particular setting. In less-optimal physical settings, staff attitudes and actions can compensate for much that is lacking to create a therapeutic and comfortable environment. Many adult day centers start out in whatever space is available, such as church basements, education buildings, or spare rooms in social services agencies. One adult day center began in a single room in a grade school building that was being renovated and used as a cultural heritage center. Nothing in the physical environment, using the most generous interpretation, could be described as warm, inviting, fun, or supportive of functioning. Yet in interviews with clients and families, those terms were used to describe the program. Clearly, staff were able to overcome the deficits of the physical environment to create an atmosphere and culture that was valued by families and clients. Lyman (1993) found that although staff could compensate for elements lacking in the physical environment, the effort to do so increased the stress experienced by the staff.

It is a commonly accepted belief that working with people with dementia is difficult and inevitably leads to burnout and high staff turnover. Yet in some care settings there is high staff morale and retention. Lyman (1993) found that staff stress and frustration decrease in organizations with policies and practices that increase staff control and provide support for staff in physical environments that decrease demand on staff. Although Lyman's research focused on adult day centers, the findings are probably equally true for air traffic controllers and factory workers. It is critically important to separate out and address the causes of staff stress and frustration in any setting and not to automatically assign the challenges of working with people with dementia as the primary cause of staff stress. Good environmental design not only facilitates functioning of the person with dementia but it also frees staff time and energy for more critical activities such as validating interactions.

Although a well-designed physical environment that supports function is a critical component of any facility, it is the interaction of the people within the space, that is, the social and cultural environments, that make the facility work for people with dementia and their families. After one family visited a newly constructed long-term care facility, they reported that it was obvious that the facility's designers were skillful in creating warm, cheerful, and functional spaces. The locked dementia care unit was especially beautiful. Each bedroom was arranged to be homelike and was decorated differently from the next, with inviting and harmonizing colors. Both the activity room and the dining room were beautiful, with warm, attractive wallpaper, comfortable furnishings, and large windows overlooking well-landscaped, attractive garden areas. The physical environment made one want to curl up in one of the many comfortable chairs with a cup of tea.

The family reported being surprised that all of the residents were lined up on one side of the hallway in wheelchairs, geri-chairs, or chairs that had been pulled out of rooms. All of the staff were at the nurses' station, and there was literally no interaction or activity on the unit outside the station. The faces of the residents reflected the isolation of their situation rather than the warmth and cheerfulness of the decor. Despite all of the thought, effort, and expense that went into the physical design of the unit, the family believed that even the ambulatory residents felt uncomfortable using the space in ways that reflected that this facility was where they lived. The unit's staff did not appear to understand the importance of social interaction for people with dementia, and neither did the assistant administrator, who was leading the tour of the facility. This experience vividly illustrates the importance of the human component of the environment and cultural context of care.

## RECOGNIZING THE IMPACT OF THE CULTURAL ENVIRONMENT

Much attention has been paid to the physical environment, but much less attention has focused on the social environment that is a natural outgrowth of the established culture. Often, care provision is considered to occur in a dyad—the person providing care and the person needing care. This limited view ignores the influence of the system and context of care, such as a family or a group care setting. Family theorists have long emphasized the influence of the whole family system on the actions of individual family members (Weeks & L'Abate, 1982). Every family constructs its own culture, including beliefs, power structure, and behavioral norms, which must be recognized to understand how the family functions. In the same way one must recognize the culture (beliefs, power structure, and behavioral norms) of any group care setting to understand the reactions of the people within the organizational system. Recognizing that every care setting, like every family, creates its own culture helps one to understand the variation among care settings. This realization also provides direction for the creation of a positive cultural environment for both staff and people with dementia.

## Beliefs

·If one accepts the premise that beliefs are the basis of attitudes and actions and even for the development of any culture, then even seemingly disparate actions in an organization are understandable. Chapter Three explored beliefs about the person with dementia as a basis for developing a framework for providing care. The beliefs that are the underpinnings of the culture in a care setting are more encompassing and include not just the people with dementia, the effects of the disease, and the care provided but also beliefs about the people providing care and the purpose of the organization. For example, the phrase "our staff are our most important resource" is heard commonly, but it is clear from observing staff functioning that the real belief is that staff must be closely supervised to enforce expectations. Several management theorists who spearheaded the management revolution of the 1980s started by changing beliefs about people, including such "new" ideas as employees can enjoy working; employees can have ideas about how to improve what is being done; and employees can be committed, contributing members of a team (Deming, 1982; Peters, 1987). Acceptance of Deming's and Peters's beliefs as a basis of action has been very slow in health care, especially in long-term care settings.

Despite the revolutionary change in manufacturing and service organizations in the 1980s, relatively few changes took place in the health care industry until the mid-1990s, and the changes that did occur were cosmetic. The "personnel department" became "human resources," care teams were established that mirrored the rigidity of the organizational structure, and there was little actual input from individuals who were placed lower in the organizational hierarchy. The health care industry is struggling to move away from this organizational model, and the move is far from complete. However, there is significant reason for hope because the market forces of the late 1990s demand that organizations change in order to survive.

Changes in how long-term care is provided, including the development of adult day services, assisted living, and adult foster homes, are helping to transform the traditional belief system. The foundation of many of these care settings is based on a different set of beliefs from those held in traditional long-term care settings. The market-driven focus on the consumer requires organizations to adopt a different set of beliefs about the person with dementia, which affects the power structure and behavioral norms of everyone in the system, both people with dementia and facility staff.

## Power Structure

Traditionally in health care settings the power structure has been hierarchical, with rigid control mechanisms. The division of labor and roles is very specifically defined; much is even mandated by law. Decision making and control of power is a top-down management model. Status is based on a person's position within the hierarchy. This organizational model is based on the Theory X assumptions of human nature—people do not want to work and must be carefully controlled and supervised to ensure that a task is completed. Because management time was consumed by so much "controlling," the span of that control or how many people one person could supervise was limited to five or six (McGregor, 1960). People who spent the most time with the object of the effort, the patient or resident, were the lowest rung of the organizational power structure ladder. Until the 1990s, this organizational model was so entrenched in American culture that many health care consumers meekly left their autonomy at the door and acquiesced to the paternalistic way in which care was provided. Many people with dementia and their family members are no longer willing to accept care that does not affirm the person.

As our knowledge increases, we need to change not only what we do but also how we do it. Organizational structure greatly influences whether or how well knowledge can be fully translated into practice. If care is not static, then the organization must be more fluid than it was in the past. Multidisciplinary teams are being touted as one of the primary mechanisms for success in health care settings in the 1990s. What being a member of a multidisciplinary team means differs from organization to organization, however. Some teams are merely collections of individuals with different expertise working on a specific problem or situation. Imagine the responsibilities in a setting or a task as a pie chart. In some care settings, team members are responsible only for their piece of the pie, usually related to the member's area of expertise. This is sufficient in some settings but not in dementia care settings. When the whole dementia care team shares the same values and goals, team members become an integral part of the power structure. Each team member is responsible for the whole pie and is accountable to other members of the team, as illustrated in Figure 7-1.

On many multidisciplinary teams, members retain fairly rigid roles (e.g., nurses do the functional assessment, activity staff conduct field trips, social workers assess the family's level of stress). This model is quite restrictive and does not work well when applied to caring for people with dementia. People, especially older adults with dementia, do not experience problems according to staff members' discipline; they just experience problems and want someone to help them. Teams that blend responsibilities tend to be much more effective in caring for people with dementia. Ruth Von Behren, a pioneer in adult day services, advocated blurring staff roles to meet clients' needs most appropriately and effectively. This approach does not mean

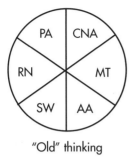
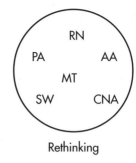

"Old" thinking                Rethinking

Figure 7-1.  Evolving team paradigms. (PA, program assistant; CNA, certified nursing assistant; RN, registered nurse; MT, music therapist; SW, social worker; AA, administrative assistant.)

that standards of safe professional practice are abandoned or that, for example, an activity staff member assumes responsibility for changing surgical dressings. Blurring roles does mean that if a person gets a paper cut during an activity, the activity staff applies a bandage. It means that the facility's bus driver is expected to notice that the wife of a client with dementia seems especially tense when he is picked up in the morning and to report this so that other staff can inquire whether assistance is needed. Because the primary focus of the team is to be supportive of the person with dementia, it is the responsibility of all staff to be alert to the many needs of and changes in function in the person and to know when to involve other members of the team.

Team members are involved in making decisions that affect the organization, such as what care approaches to implement or use, how care is organized, and who to hire. Because each person brings unique skills, abilities, interests, and experiences to the team, respect for these differing abilities encourages team members to learn from and rely on one another. More than the number of staff members, the way that care is provided and how the workday is organized are most critical. A nurse can assess functional ability, swollen ankles, level of alertness, and much else while leading a reminiscence group. Each person on the staff can and should help with the entire range of activities, from groups to activities of daily living. Each person's professional background and experience provides a particular way of assessing a situation. When these differing perspectives are shared in staff meetings, they provide a richer assessment of the person. In addition, they are more responsive to the person with dementia. For example, if a person's pants are wet, he or she may be embarrassed. For a staff member to say, "Let me get someone to help you," only adds to the embarrassment. It is more comforting to have someone say, "I know where your clothes are. Let's go get into some dry ones now."

## Behavioral Norms

Beliefs that are common to the members of any system are incorporated by those individuals and become the basis of behaviors in a specific circumstance. These behavioral norms are reinforced formally through the organization's power structure and informally through peer pressure. As beliefs about the person with dementia change from viewing the person as an "empty shell" to a person with abilities and impairments, the behavioral norms of how care is provided also will change. The challenge for members of the system is to mold the change in ways that are helpful rather than detrimental to the person with dementia. As it becomes more commonly accepted that care for a person with dementia is expected to accomplish a goal, there is a danger that a rehabilitation model of care could be adopted. In the rehabilitation model the role of staff is to help the person improve, but the responsibility for the actual work of improvement resides with the person with the impairment. It is clear that this model of care is not appropriate for people with dementia. A palliative model of care, adopted by the hospice movement, seems more appropriate. The goal of a palliative model is to mitigate the impact of the disease, but the responsibility for the mitigation resides with the person providing care, not with the person with the illness.

If each member of the team clearly understands, internalizes, and takes action to validate the person with dementia, then the care environment also should foster a sense of well-being for both the person with dementia and members of the team. This sort of culture usually does not occur by happenstance but grows out of the creation of a team approach to care that is based on personal responsibility to use one's skills to contribute to the team's goals and on accountability for one's actions. Because team members learn from one another, individual abilities are valued and create an environment that supports personal and professional growth. Helping staff to develop skills both formally and informally enriches the program because the more diverse the skills and interests of the staff, the more likely the organization is to implement programming that will meet the diverse interests and abilities of people with dementia.

# *R*ethinking in Practice ················································································

*Assessing the culture of an environment*

*To understand any culture, family, or organization, we must look at the whole system. The actions of people within the organization often provide more insight about the beliefs that are the basis of the organization than do the written mission statement and philosophy. As one director of a facility explained, "They (the administration) don't want to spend any money on staff training, but they spend huge amounts on the interior design. They say the resident is the primary focus of what we do, but it's really marketing to the families that's important to them."*

*Consider the specific ways that staff interact with colleagues and with people with dementia. Describe the beliefs that these interactions convey.*

In what ways are these beliefs affirming (or not) of staff and of people with dementia?

How do the conveyed beliefs fit with your beliefs about your peers and people with dementia?

What changes in elements of the organizational structure would help to provide more effective care for people with dementia?

If staff are expected to try new ideas and activities, then management must expect that some will not work very well. When an activity is unsuccessful, it is important for the team to thoughtfully consider the reasons it did not work, instead of blame a staff member or avoid the activity in the future. In staff meetings in which each team member's ideas and contributions are valued, staff share successes, work out problems, and learn from one another. Staff attitudes and actions are of primary importance in the creation of a culture that is supportive of the person with dementia. Staff who do not feel supported and validated by management are less likely to be supportive of a person with dementia. Sharing information among team members also is important because if staff are expected to be supportive of the person with dementia, they must know that person. If staff are expected to use a person's long-term memories and sense of self in choosing appropriate care approaches, they must know about the person. As information about a person with dementia is learned, it must be shared with all members of the team.

## BLENDING ENVIRONMENTAL COMPONENTS INTO A THERAPEUTIC MILIEU

When determining how best to provide care for the person with dementia, we must consider all of the components of the environment. Together the components form a framework for the provision of care that supports the functional abilities of the person and compensates for his or her losses. In addition to considering the components of a therapeutic milieu, we need to consider ways to combine these components in ways that support the abilities of the person with dementia. *Milieu* is a term that is used in psychiatric care settings because the importance of the totality of one's experience is recognized. The concept is essential in caring for people with dementia because all of the elements of the environment interact and blend to form a whole that determines the kinds of experiences that the person will have.

Until the 1990s the reductionist focus of the health care industry emphasized how care was provided rather than how it was experienced by the person receiving care. The industry now acknowledges that it is the quality of life of people with dementia (with the focus on what is experienced by the person with dementia) rather than the quality of the care provided (with the focus on what is done by the staff) that is truly important. Although the provision and experience of care are intertwined, our focus must center on the experience of the person with dementia. Gunderson (1983) described five elements in a therapeutic milieu, which were adapted by Taft, Delaney, Seman, and Stansell (1993) to describe an environment for providing care in which the person with dementia experiences safety, structure, support, involvement, and validation.

## Safety

In Blaser's unpublished paper, *Zen and the Art of Quality* (1987), she emphasized that although the perceptions of quality in caring vary dramatically, safety is perceived by everyone as a basic need. If safety is considered to be the maintenance of physical well-being and the prevention of dangerous or self-destructive actions, then we can easily agree that it is probably a basic requirement for anyone, especially for people with dementia (Taft et al., 1993). The challenge for staff is to provide safety in a way that is not aggressive or presumptuous. Staff need to be in control of a situation, but they must do it in a way that is not perceived as controlling by the person they are trying to assist.

The therapeutic milieu, or the blending of the physical, social, and cultural environments, can be created to meet safety needs in many ways. For example, access to areas that could pose a danger can be limited and people can be engaged in activities so that they are not constantly being told, "No," "Stop," or, "You can't go in there." We can ask a gentleman, "May I take your arm so you can escort me down this sidewalk?" rather than lead him by his hand or forearm so that he does not walk away from the group. We are in physical contact with the person and meeting his or her safety needs, but the first approach also preserves the person's dignity.

All of us have experienced the impact that an environment can have, generating feelings of safety or insecurity. Many people with dementia live with profound feelings of insecurity and need an environment that promotes a sense of mastery and safety. The following situation illustrates this point.

> Mel returned to a group care setting after surgery to repair a broken hip. He seemed a bit more confused than usual and was using a wheelchair to limit the amount of stress on his hip until healing was complete. After lunch one day, he asked to be taken to the bathroom. The staff member moved the wheelchair close to the commode and assisted Mel to stand. When she offered to help and began unzipping his pants, he began to hit her and shout, "Help!" Another staff person responding to the commotion saw that Mel was not only highly agitated but that his attempts to hit the staff person were endangering his tenuous ability to stand. To prevent another fall, she supported him from behind and with another staff member reseated him in the wheelchair. Attempts to calm Mel were fruitless, and he continued to scream and attempt to hit both of the staff members. It took other staff more than an hour to calm him. This behavior, which was so out of character for Mel, was puzzling to staff because later he asked to "go pee" and urinated without incident.
>
> The next day after lunch, Mel again asked to be taken to the bathroom. As a staff member wheeled him past the sink to position the wheelchair close to the commode, Mel said, "Whoa!" and held his hands out toward the sink. Only then did staff begin to understand his behavior the previous day: When he asked to go to the bathroom, he had wanted only to wash his hands. When the staff member began to undress him, he may have felt that he was being assaulted and responded by defending himself. In some settings Mel's behavior would be considered simply a "catastrophic reaction," without an attempt being made to understand the reason behind the behavior. The staff, out of concern for Mel's physical safety, understood that they had disregarded his need for emotional safety and learned from the experience.

Sometimes families express concern that a loved one with dementia does not want to wear a Safe Return bracelet (an Alzheimer's Association program). Out of concern for the person's safety needs, a person's emotional needs may be disregarded. Sensitive to their mother's pride, one family knew that simply telling her "You have to wear this now for your own safety" would not be acceptable. Instead, they wrapped the bracelet as a gift and the grandchildren presented it to her at a family dinner. She not only wore the bracelet willingly but she also often described it as "a gift from those sweet grandchildren of mine." Knowing the person with dementia is a primary determinant in deciding what approach will be the most effective in a specific situation to help the person feel safe and be safe.

## Structure

Structure is furnished for the person with dementia by other people who provide temporal landmarks, a routine that provides predictability in the person's day, and by the physical environment (Taft et al., 1993). It is difficult to imagine how perplexing and possibly even frightening a situation can be when a person with dementia has lost his or her concept of time and everything is in the "now." Alan Lightman's book *Einstein's Dreams* (1994), which explores the different ways that people respond to time, provides some provocative insights into what life must be like for people with dementia as the disease progresses. In one dream, none of the people in a city have any long-term memory or sense of time and therefore have knowledge only of the present. Some people create a "Book of Life" in which they write events

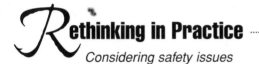

## ethinking in Practice

*Considering safety issues*

*In providing care for people with dementia, some caregivers exhibit a "we/they" attitude, based on the belief that those caring for a person with dementia do not share the same basic needs or feelings as a person with dementia. Actions arising from this belief can and do lead to contentious relationships between the people providing care and the people receiving care, especially about issues of safety. Attention to the feelings of the person with dementia is essential because the feeling of safety is as important as being safe.*

*If you were in your living room and heard someone scream, "Help me!" what would your response be? If you recognized the voice, would you be concerned about the person? Would you see if you could help? If you did not recognize the voice, would you be frightened?*

*Consider the response of a person with dementia who is sitting in the living room of a group care facility when hearing someone scream, "Help me!"*

If the person with dementia exhibits concern, what are some possible staff responses?
If the person with dementia exhibits fear, what are some possible staff responses?
Have you ever heard a staff member respond by telling the person with dementia to ignore the screams because "it's just Rosie, and she screams all the time"? Is this response likely to provide reassurance or increase the person's fear and concern? What are some potential responses of a person with dementia to this approach?

as they happen, so that they can know themselves and their history. There is a sense of a desperate need for structure for these people and a fearfulness of losing a feeling of connectedness to their past. Other people who "have learned to live in a world without memory" have quit writing in or even reading their "Book of Life" and simply relish each moment and find meaning in the present (Lightman, 1994).

Those of us who have had the opportunity to work with older adults with dementia have known people who responded in both ways described by Lightman, as well as some who responded in-between these ways. Their responses have made us aware of the variability in the kind and amount of structure that may be helpful to people with dementia. For some who want and need structure and information, calendars marking the days, notes about coming events, and pictures and verbal reminders of past accomplishments and relationships are critically important. For other people, this sort of "reality orientation" is confusing and distressing. We need to be sensitive to the kind and amount of structure that is helpful. For example, Ruth, a lady of great wisdom who has Alzheimer's disease, eloquently explained this need for sensitivity. Her activity group was discussing a person who had just left the room seeming very confused. Several group members expressed concern about the person, and a staff member asked what they thought might help her. Ruth said, "Everybody gets confused, but it's not the same for everyone. You have to know what's confusing and what kind of help that person will accept. Each of us need help in a different way."

For some people with dementia who have lost the ability to structure time, the structure of program activities provides temporal landmarks that are comforting. The routine of the day provides some predictability, a sense of rhythm, and famil-

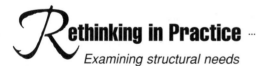

# $\mathcal{R}$ethinking in Practice

### Examining structural needs

*When we think of structural ways to lessen a person's confusion, typically we think of signs that help with wayfinding or pictures that remind the person or family of past accomplishments. As we have learned more about how people with Alzheimer's disease actually experience the illness, we have learned that temporal landmarks and program structure can reduce the confusion that is experienced. Learning to identify what is confusing and distressing to a person with dementia often is challenging for a person providing care, but success is one of the rewards that make working with people with dementia a joy.*

*Think about a person with dementia who is confused and distressed. Consider what is confusing to him or her:*

Is something in the physical environment contributing to his or her confusion?
Could the person have misperceived something that he or she heard, saw, or smelled?
Does the person seem not to understand what is expected of him or her?
Could a treatable sensory loss, such as cataracts, be contributing to the person's confusion?
What are other possible causes of the person's confusion and distress?
What approaches might minimize the person's confusion?

iarity. The physical environment can provide cues about what kind of actions are appropriate. The single most frequently asked question in adult day centers is, "When am I going home?" Concern about going home is quite understandable because many people with dementia may not remember where home is or how to get there. The anxiety level in people with dementia in adult day centers increases considerably during the afternoon. Because some adult day centers understand these feelings of anxiety and individuals' abilities to respond appropriately to environmental cues, they schedule a chapel service in the afternoon, just before people begin to go home. For many people the familiarity of the service is comforting and the setting is reassuring—people always go home after a church service.

## Support

Taft and colleagues (1993) described support as conscious efforts to help people feel understood and to enhance their self-esteem. It is important to note that these are conscious efforts, not just happenstance. Nissenboim and Vroman (1998) emphasized the need for intentionality and stressed the importance of creating opportunities for people with dementia to feel competent and supported through activities that are appropriate to their remaining abilities. Making a conscious effort means that programs that provide care for people with dementia do not rely solely on the innate empathy and caring of staff but also emphasize the importance of thoughtful planning of activities and taking deliberate steps to develop supportive relationships. It is the responsibility of caregivers to create a milieu in which people with dementia feel supported by building supportive relationships and recognizing the supportive relationships that are created between people with dementia.

The most important aspect of being supportive is communication, both verbal and nonverbal; that is, not just what is said but the way it is said. Research in the field of psychology has found that 90% of all human communication is nonverbal (Mehrabian, 1981). Humans have an enormous capacity both to express thoughts and feelings and to understand the thoughts and feelings of others nonverbally. Usually, our nonverbal communication rather than our verbal communication conveys empathy and support or lack of these feelings. Our manner, tone of voice, and facial expressions vividly convey our actual feelings and sometimes are not congruent with our words. Making conscious efforts to be supportive means that we pay close attention to what we are communicating in both words and actions. The people who are effective in establishing relationships with people with dementia are not just naturally kind and empathic but also thoughtful about the ways that caring and supportive feelings are expressed. There is a conscious intent, followed by skillful communication.

Although paying attention to what we are communicating is essential, the primary focus of communication with a person with dementia should be on understanding what that person is expressing rather than getting him or her to do what we want. We want to support a person's feeling of competence and for him or her to know that he or she has communicated feelings and wishes, even if most of the verbal skills have been lost. Sharing with people with dementia how they positively affect our lives also is critical to developing a relationship that is supportive and validating.

Although conscious effort is an essential element in consistently conveying support, for most people support means "not having to go it alone." The need to be with people who understand one's experiences and feelings has led to the creation of a wide variety of support groups based on the concept of peer support (e.g., Alcoholics Anonymous, caregiver support groups). It is generally recognized that peer support is helpful to some people early in the course of Alzheimer's disease. However, the capacity of people to be supportive of others throughout the illness is not well acknowledged. Experience in working with people throughout the course of the disease has provided ample evidence of this capacity to relate to others in distress in comforting ways.

## Involvement

Involvement has been described as engaging or interacting with the social environment (Taft et al., 1993). As social beings, we need to relate to others meaningfully. We need to share our joys, our troubles, and the ordinary "stuff" of life. Although obviously people with dementia experience the same kinds of social needs as people without dementia, sometimes we become so focused on the mechanics of providing care that we lose sight of the reality experienced by people with dementia. For example, while the director of a dementia care unit was meeting with a faculty physician to arrange observational visits for residents in internal medicine, a group of people with dementia returned from a walk. One of the women had picked up a beer bottle during her walk and was looking for a place to dispose of it. As the director took the bottle to put it in the recycle bin, she winked at the woman with de-

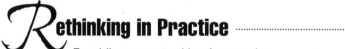

## $\mathcal{R}$ethinking in Practice

*Providing opportunities for ongoing support*

*Although support groups are important for some people with dementia, meeting a person's need for support should not be relegated to a designated group. All interactions need to be supportive of a person's sense of self, provide the opportunity for him or her to freely express feelings (positive and negative), and validate that the person has been understood. Think about the ways that you receive support from others in your personal life.*

Do you find support primarily in formal or informal interactions?
What is the nature and location of the interactions that are the most supportive?

*Consider ways to provide this feeling of support to someone with dementia.*

What are some ways to create or use day-to-day interactions to convey a feeling of support?
What nonverbal ways express support for the person?

mentia and said, teasingly, "I thought you were going for a walk in the park, not to a bar. Isn't it a little early in the day?" They shared a laugh at the thought of this very proper lady in a bar at midmorning. After the woman left the room, the physician confessed to the director, "I didn't know that they could still laugh." This comment is especially sad considering that this physician was responsible for educating others and held such a constricted view of people with dementia.

As Alzheimer's disease progresses, many people become less inhibited and lose some of their characteristic reserve about expressing feelings, both positive and negative. As a person's social facade fades, he or she is able to interact with others in more genuine and authentic ways than before onset of the disease. For example, Ruby often made wry, witty, and on-target comments about situations and others around her. One day a staff member shared with Ruby's daughter, Elaine, some bits of Ruby's "wit and wisdom." Elaine said that as her mother became more disinhibited, Elaine understood her better. It seemed that throughout Elaine's life, her mother had been very reserved and rarely shared her thoughts or feelings. As she lost this reticence, she was able to make her wishes well known despite the language impairments caused by the disease, and Elaine was able to connect with her in a whole new way. Elaine believed that their relationship was enhanced rather than diminished by Alzheimer's disease. There is a "realness" with people with dementia that can be enriching to others around them. Being with people with dementia gives us an opportunity to share moments of joy, wit, and poignancy in ways that enhance our lives. The reciprocity in relationships with people with dementia is sometimes overlooked or even discounted as the person's language skills diminish.

These enriching and reciprocal relationships can occur only if the people providing care recognize the social needs of the person with dementia and accept the responsibility to meet those needs. Sabat (1998) emphasized that a person with dementia must have the cooperation of others to help express his or her social identity.

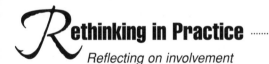

# ethinking in Practice

*Reflecting on involvement*

*If we accept the view that "persons exist in relationships; interdependence is a necessary condition of being human" (Kitwood & Bredin, 1992, p. 270), then we are able to develop an appreciation of the impact of the connection and interaction on us and the people around us, including those with dementia.*

*Reflect on the elements in a therapeutic milieu that encourage people with dementia to become involved and interact with others. What are some elements that discourage this behavior? Consider the ways that your own life has been enriched by having a relationship with people with dementia.*

*Keep a notebook handy to jot down reflections on the times when you feel really connected to a person with dementia. Think about the following:*

What did you bring to the interaction or experience?
What did you gain from the interaction or experience?

Clinical experience has demonstrated that even people with severe cognitive impairment still have a sense of self that is reinforced or is not reinforced by those around them.

## Validation

Validation is a process that affirms a person's individuality, feelings, and abilities. Behaviors are seen as meaningful and a way of communicating rather than as problems (Taft et al., 1993). Both family and professionals caring for a person with dementia frequently described repetitive questions and behaviors as problems. For example, people with memory loss may ask repetitive questions, which can be frustrating for the caregiver and may lead to being short-tempered with the person. If we understand that the person does not remember asking the question before and does not remember the answer, then we can provide the answer with less frustration. An even better alternative is to identify the need that the person is trying to express and find a way to respond to that need.

Several years ago, Jane Stansell learned firsthand what it must be like for the person who does not remember asking repetitive questions and who gets a short or aggravated response. The day after the Chicago Bulls basketball team won their second world championship, a friend asked her to buy him a cap with the "Back to Back" logo. Late in the afternoon, she stopped at a department store to pick up the hat. She entered the store through the linens department and asked an employee who was straightening towels, "Where is the Bulls' stuff?" The employee responded, very curtly, "Downstairs." Jane apologized for interrupting her work and went on her way, feeling chastised and confused. On later reflection she realized that even though it was the first time that she had asked the question, the employee must have answered the same question several hundred times that day. Jane also realized that people with dementia must experience similar feelings many times every day, perceiving that an action was somehow inappropriate but not knowing why.

Asking repetitive questions may be a sign of anxiety rather than a simple forgetting of the answer or the question. Under such circumstances, responding to each repetitive question may increase the level of anxiety rather than diminish it. Anxiety in the person with dementia may be reduced if we can engage the person in an activity or task that diverts his or her attention from the repetitive questioning. Our understanding of the person and the reason behind the repetitive questions determine whether we give a person a note providing information or engage him or her in a task, such as polishing silver, folding napkins, sanding wood, or taking a walk. The goal of each approach is to help the person maintain a sense of control in the situation, facilitate the use of strengths to solve or cope with the problem being experienced, and validate the person's worth.

Providing a milieu that validates the individuality of a person with dementia requires the development of a program that consistently affirms his or her unique abilities. Validation is not just provided by others but also is the result of experiencing success in one's daily activities. Programming that is designed to utilize the person's retained skills and abilities provides multiple opportunities for validation. For instance, the person who has played the piano daily since childhood may retain this skill far into the illness. Opportunities to use this ability for the enjoyment of others can be validating for the musician. As with any retained skill, one needs to be aware of the degree of retained skill and fit the task to the ability. For example, Edith may retain the ability to remember a number of popular songs and the musical ability to accompany a group sing-along. Jaime, who has significant cognitive impairment, retains his musical ability but frequently forgets that he has played the chorus and plays it several times before moving on to the next verse, or he plays another song, making it difficult for others to sing along. Instead of asking him to play for a group sing-along, he is asked to play while others have coffee after lunch, so that people can take a moment to relax and enjoy the music.

Most people have a need to be active and useful. Although almost everyone enjoys leisure activities, not many people relish the idea of a lifetime of cruise ship–type activities. In addition to having fun, people with dementia need opportunities to feel as though their contributions count. In 1993 severe flooding of the Mississippi River threatened many southern Illinois towns. Sandbagging became a primary concern, and many citizens of these towns spent days and nights building dikes. Adult day center clients who were frail or had cognitive impairments were concerned about the flooding and decided that they could help by cutting strings for

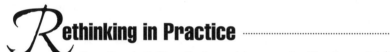

## ethinking in Practice

*Creating activities that provide opportunities for validation*

*The unique strengths and needs of each person with dementia must be considered individually, understanding that our approach not only may be different for each person but also may vary depending on the person's functional ability at any given time. "Fuzzy logic" is a popular topic among mathematicians and designers of many consumer electronics products (Kosko, 1993). The basic premise of fuzzy logic is that few situations are clearly black or white, either one thing or the other. Fuzzy logic has been used to develop "smart machines," such as razors that assess the density and thickness of a beard and make adjustments to provide a comfortable, close shave. Because people have infinitely more creative capacity than smart machines, we should be able to develop activities and approaches that use the varying abilities and accommodate the needs of the person with dementia. Consider the retained skills and strengths of a person with dementia and ask yourself the following questions:*

What kinds of activities can be provided to use each of these skills?
Are some approaches more effective than others in engaging the person?
What is the person's response to the activity?
How does this response differ from his or her response when he or she did not have the skills necessary to successfully complete an activity?
Are there ways that the activity program can be changed to optimize the opportunity for validation?

the sandbags. This activity gave them an opportunity to make a valuable contribution to their community. There are many opportunities in everyday life for people with dementia to contribute—helping to set the table for lunch, pushing someone's wheelchair, or holding their own shirt while being changed.

## PROVIDING A SUPPORTIVE MILIEU FOR EACH PERSON WITH DEMENTIA

As mentioned previously, behaviors that are exhibited by people with dementia are too often regarded as a problem to be managed rather than as a response to something in the environment or lacking in it. The example that follows brings together many of the concepts described in this chapter to show how a milieu can be developed that is supportive of an individual with dementia: After being discharged from an adult day center because she consistently exhibited "verbally and physically aggressive and abusive behavior," Eva was admitted to another center. At the second adult day center, Eva exhibited none of the behaviors that had been so problematic at the first. When staff from the first center visited the second center, they were amazed at the difference in her behavior. She participated in activities in a very pleasant and friendly manner. In discussing the differences in Eva's behavior, the staff from the first center said that the differences in the environments of the two centers mirrored the differences in Eva's behavior. They offered that perhaps her actions were different because of the difference in the environments.

In discussing these environmental differences staff quickly became aware that many factors contributed to the changes in Eva's actions. The cultures of the two centers were very different—beliefs about people with dementia, the meaning behind their behavior, and the purpose of care differed significantly. The leadership and staff at the second center were strongly committed to the belief that it is possible for the care of people with dementia to mitigate the impact of the disease on their functioning and social interactions. The staff at the second center believed it was critical to know Eva as a person. At 86, Eva was still in many ways the matriarch of her family, with a strong sense of propriety and a long history as a stern disciplinarian. She had worked hard to support her family and had little time or appreciation for leisure and recreational activities. Because staff understood these facts about Eva, they made a conscientious effort to affirm Eva's view of herself, and they understood that they, not Eva, must make changes. The young men on staff came to realize that Eva considered it disrespectful for men to wear hats inside, so they were always careful to remove their caps when in a room with her.

Eva was easily distracted and responded very negatively to noisy environments. The physical design of the second center made it possible to organize activities in rooms that limited distractions. The telephones were programmed not to ring, the small scale of the rooms limited the number of people in them to 15 or 20, and furniture was arranged to focus attention and facilitate interaction. The bathrooms were located close to the activity room and were equipped with directional signs so that Eva could go to the bathroom independently, despite her difficulties with walking and wayfinding.

The social environment of the second center also was quite different. The staff understood the importance of interpersonal interaction as a way of validating a person with dementia. Staff actions demonstrated the belief that Eva retained her core identity, or personhood, throughout the course of the disease. However, the impairment caused by the disease required others to help mitigate the impact of the disease on Eva's ability to relate to others socially. Because the amount of support or mitigation varies among people and within a person, it was necessary to determine carefully the amount of support that was provided. This level of individual support is difficult to provide in a heterogeneous setting; therefore, Eva was clustered into a group with others who had similar abilities and needs. Clustering made it possible for staff to match her individual needs without arranging for a one-to-one interaction ratio.

The physical, social, and cultural environments were adapted to support Eva's specific strengths and abilities and to compensate for her specific losses by eliminating, to the extent possible, all of the barriers that prevented her from using her retained skills. All of the components of the therapeutic milieu were adjusted, to the extent possible, to be supportive of the person Eva knew herself to be. In addition, all of the elements of the milieu were blended together to create a culture of care that fostered the feeling of well-being of a person with dementia.

## REFERENCES

Alzheimer's Association. (1997). *The key elements of dementia care*. Chicago: Author.
Blaser, J. (1987, October). *Zen and the art of quality*. Paper presented at the Illinois Governor's Conference for Aging Network, Chicago.
Brawley, E.C. (1997). *Designing for Alzheimer's disease: Strategies for creating better care environments*. New York: John Wiley & Sons.
Calkins, M. (1988). *Design for dementia*. Owings Mills, MD: National Health Publishing.
Cohen, U., & Weisman, G. (1991). *Holding on to home*. Baltimore: The Johns Hopkins University Press.
Deming, W.E. (1982). *Out of crisis*. Cambridge: Massachusetts Institute of Technology, Center for Advanced Engineering Study.
Erdman, D. (Ed.). (1982). *The complete poetry and prose of William Blake* (p. 36). Garden City, NJ: Anchor Books.
Gunderson, J.G. (1983). An overview of modern milieu therapy. In J.G. Gunderson, O.A. Will, & L.R. Mosher (Eds.), *Principles and practices of milieu therapy* (pp. 1–13). New York: Jason Aronson.
Kitwood, T., & Bredin, K. (1992). Towards a theory of dementia care: Personhood and well being. *Ageing and Society, 12*, 269–287.
Kosko, B. (1993). *Fuzzy thinking*. New York: Hyperion.
Lightman, A. (1994). *Einstein's dreams*. New York: Warner Books.
Lyman, K.A. (1993). *Day in, day out with Alzheimer's: Stress in caregiving relationships*. Philadelphia: Temple University Press.

McGregor, D. (1960). *The human side of enterprise.* New York: McGraw-Hill.

Mehrabian, A. (1981). *Silent messages.* Belmont, CA: Wadsworth.

Namazi, K., & Johnson, B. (1991, November/December). Physical environmental cues to reduce the problems of incontinence in Alzheimer's disease units. *American Journal of Alzheimer's Care and Research,* 22–28.

Nissenboim, S., & Vroman, C. (1998). *The positive interactions program of activities for people with Alzheimer's disease.* Baltimore: Health Professions Press.

Peters, T.J. (1987). *Thriving on chaos: Handbook for a management revolution.* New York: Alfred P. Knopf.

Sabat, S. (1998). Voices of Alzheimer's disease sufferers: A call for treatment based on personhood. *Journal of Clinical Ethics, 9*(1), 35–48.

Taft, L., Delaney, K., Seman, D., & Stansell, J. (1993, October). Dementia care: Creating a therapeutic milieu. *Journal of Gerontological Nursing,* 30–39.

Weeks, G., & L'Abate, L. (1982). *Paradoxical psychotherapy.* New York: Brunner/Mazel.

# $\mathcal{R}$edesigning Care Programs

*You can complain because roses have thorns, or you can rejoice because thorns have roses.*

*Ziggy*

If we accept the premise proposed by many clinicians that everything a person does is an activity, we can identify ways to shape individual interactions and the milieu to validate a person with dementia. Although this is sometimes challenging, it can be even more challenging in a group setting to address the diversity of abilities and needs of people with dementia. In group care settings the program design must bring together all elements of the environment—physical, social, and cultural—to foster a feeling of well-being for each person.

It is almost impossible in a group setting to create a single activity or program space that provides the opportunity for involvement and validation for everyone. This is confirmed both in the everyday experience of clinicians and in research such as Neugarten's (1988) findings about the diversity among older adults, which vividly demonstrate that the range of knowledge, experiences, abilities, interests, and needs are more diverse than in any other age group. Understanding the need to provide a range of activities and programming led those caring for groups of older people to develop "parallel programming" for the people with dementia in a given group (Silcox & Cohen, 1987).

As awareness of the unique needs of people with dementia evolved, specialized programs were developed. This approach to care made possible many advances in the provision of care for people with dementia; however, it was not a panacea. Although this step in the development of programming was appropriate for people with dementia, it became apparent that there was too much diversity in the range of people's abilities and impairments for a single approach, activity, or environment to be universally effective. The person who has an attention span of 5 minutes is not able to participate in an activity for 30 minutes, no matter how interesting the activity or how much pleasure that activity brought in the past. This is frustrating for the person with the short attention span, and the need for constant redirection

**113**

disrupts the flow of the group activity, may frustrate other participants involved in the activity, and often results in some members of the group making unkind comments to or about the person. The staff member trying to lead the group is faced with a choice of constant disruption while redirecting and soothing ruffled feelings or just letting the person leave the group.

Although the person whose behavior is "disruptive" in a group setting gets attention, other people in the group may be equally disengaged, but they display the disengagement differently. People who withdraw emotionally rather than physically are not disruptive to the group process, but neither are they a part of the group. The group may be beyond some individuals' ability. Lacking the capacity to express this inability, these people often sit in the group with vacant facial expressions or sleep during an activity. For instance, as Roberto became more cognitively impaired, he seemed to experience increasing difficulty following the group discussions he had previously enjoyed. A quiet and polite person, he would "drift off" in discussion groups, and staff noted that he was sleeping more often during group sessions instead of participating as he had in the past. When he was engaged in a group with more "hands-on" activities, he began to participate actively. Other participants, who may be bored because a particular activity does not use their retained skills or pique their interest, may quietly endure the activity. For example, when Sophie described a group as a part of a program evaluation, she said, "When she [group leader] began reading poetry to us, I wondered what I had gotten myself into." Although neither Roberto nor Sophie was disruptive, some staff might simply describe their behavior as passive participation rather than explore the reasons for missed opportunities and interaction. It is much less stressful for everyone if the activity is fitted to the person instead of trying to get the person to do something that is beyond or below his or her capabilities. As clinicians began to appreciate the true diversity in the abilities and needs of people with dementia, the practice of clustering people into groups with shared characteristics has grown.

It is possible to teach a group of children, kindergarten through 12th grade, in one room, although this approach is no longer viewed as desirable. Some have difficulty concentrating while others are engaged in a different activity. Children learn better when they are clustered in groups or classes with those who have similar skills and abilities and are taught in separate rooms. Thus, the one-room schoolhouse is part of history, not of our current experience in education. A similar change must occur in the field of dementia care: We must move beyond the one-room schoolhouse approach. To enable people to participate in activities to the fullest extent possible, the activities must be strengths-based and must take into account heterogeneous skills and needs. Because "one size does not fit all," it is helpful to cluster people into groups of individuals with similar skills and needs and to develop activities based on the skills of the group.

## CLUSTERING AS A WAY TO ORGANIZE CARE

Clustering people with dementia into groups of similar abilities and needs is a way to adjust all of the components of the milieu to be supportive of the person with dementia. The physical, social, and cultural environments can be adapted to support the specific strengths and abilities of each person in a group setting. The milieu also can be designed to compensate for the specific losses of each group member by eliminating, as much as one can, the barriers that may prevent a person from using his or her retained skills.

The concept of clustering is based on the belief that people with dementia retain their essence, core identity, or personhood throughout the course of the disease. It is an extension of the way that most people live their lives. We tend to have an affinity for people with whom we share interests and abilities. As a result of the disease process, many people with dementia lose the capacity to seek others with whom they might share a rewarding and supportive relationship. Clustering is a means of compensating for that loss.

The impairments caused by the disease require the help of others to mitigate the impact of the disease on the person's physical and psychosocial functional ability, including the ability to relate to others. Because the amount of the support or mitigation varies among people, and even within a person, it is necessary to continuously assess and alter carefully the amount of support that is provided. Clustering people into groups with others who have similar abilities and needs makes supporting individual strengths and meeting individual needs possible without employing one-to-one staff–client/resident ratios.

This program design is not static but rather is a dynamic process that is responsive to the specific characteristics of each member in any group setting. The

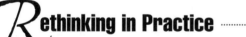

## *R*ethinking in Practice

*Considering the need to move beyond the "one-room schoolhouse" program design*

The pitfalls involved in providing care for a group of people with diverse abilities and needs present a dilemma for many clinicians. Developing ways to accommodate diverse needs and support a wide variety of strengths in a group setting is a frequent topic of conversation for those directly involved in providing care for people with dementia. It is generally recognized that the one-room schoolhouse approach to dementia care does not work, but often these discussions are focused on ways to get "problem people" to participate in planned activities.

*Think about conversations you have had with peers about these challenges.*

What were some of the frequently expressed frustrations?
What feelings do these frustrations generate in you or your peers?
What feelings about people with dementia come up?

*Consider your peers' suggestions of ways to deal with these challenging situations.*

Were the suggestions focused on individual approaches for the person who disrupted the group or ways to change the group to be more appropriate for the person?
Were suggestions focused primarily on people who disrupted the group?
Did people who quietly disengaged from groups receive an equal focus?

number of clusters depends on the characteristics of the people in a setting at a given time. There may be times when more or fewer clusters are needed to create environments that are appropriate to the varying needs of the individuals. Clustering is a means of creating a homogeneous group for the purpose of providing activities and care that are a good fit for the person with dementia. It is a means of helping a person with dementia succeed in an activity, task, or interaction.

People are clustered into groups based on current functioning ability, not interests (current or past), and these are not rigid assignments. In some settings people may spend most of their time in a specific group, and in other settings people may be part of a specific group only during planned activities. However, because many people with dementia have difficulty structuring their time, the activity programs in some group settings are quite structured, with minimal downtime. Experience has shown structure in program design to be so important that some regulatory bodies (e.g., state departments of health or aging) even mandate that a specific number of hours of structured activities during the day be provided on dementia-specific units.

## Activities within Clusters

If we think of *activity* in its broadest sense, it is easy to understand why we generally classify everything we do as an activity. This perspective, the genesis of activities of daily living (ADLs) and instrumental activities in daily living (IADLs), acknowledges that activities for the person with dementia are not just those that are organized and scheduled. A result of working within this perspective is that every staff member is an activity coordinator who is responsible for knowing each person with dementia and his or her strengths and appropriate ways to compensate for his or her losses. Every interaction is an opportunity to provide the kind of social support and relationship that is needed to help the person with dementia maintain a sense of well-being. In each homogeneous cluster, activities are developed on the basis of the interests and strengths and adapted to the specific functional abilities of the people in the group. This method provides the framework for care and opportunities for each person involved to experience success and pleasure in all activities and interactions.

Many organized activities can be successfully adapted for people with a wide range of abilities. However, it is almost impossible to make the multiple adaptations necessary for each person within a single heterogeneous group to be comfortable and successful. With homogeneous groups based on functional abilities, it is much less complex to adapt an activity so that it is appropriate for each person. Cooking treats for a special holiday is an example of an activity that may be enjoyed by many people. However, because it is unlikely that all of the people who may enjoy cooking in a specific setting have the same level of functional ability, it is often difficult to adapt a cooking group so that it is equally enjoyable for everyone.

If people are clustered into homogeneous groups, then the adaptations are less obvious to those involved and the experience is likely to be comfortable and enjoyable. People with good long-term memory are likely to remember favorite treats for specific holidays, and if their short-term memory is fairly intact they may enjoy planning and shopping for the necessary ingredients and preparing the treat. People in this group also may enjoy reminiscing about times that they prepared cookies. During the preparation, there may be lively discussions of alternative methods of preparation or ingredients. While the treats are cooking, people in this group can enjoy the anticipation of sampling the results of their efforts.

Another group of people whose long- and short-term memory are significantly impaired may enjoy making a holiday pie, with the staff doing the planning, obtaining the ingredients, and breaking down the preparation into tasks that individual group members can perform successfully. It is enjoyment and success in the process that is critical. Members of this group may not even remember their contributions to the project when the pie is cooked and served, even if they are reminded. In the group of older adults with minor impairments, the role of staff is more of a facilitator; in the group of people with significant impairment, staff have more responsibility and take a more active role in cueing and leading the activity.

Other activities, such as going on an outing to a church service or a special garden tour, may be enjoyable and appropriate for people with a wide range of abilities. Although interest is a primary criterion for the success of any activity, the ability to carry out the activity successfully is equally important. Some people, including those with dementia, enjoy going to a baseball game; others find it boring. For example, Bernice is 93, has a Mini-Mental State Examination score of 0, has little short- or long-term memory, and loves the Chicago Cubs. She still enjoys going to games at Wrigley Field. Although she does not remember what has occurred in previous innings and does not even remember that she has been to a game when she is back on the bus, she truly enjoys the ambience of being at the ballpark and shouts, "Go Cubs!" with fervor equal to any other fan. Tony is an equally ardent Cubs fan but is so easily overstimulated that the noise and confusion of the ballpark would be overwhelming and intolerable. For him, watching a game on television is a much more appropriate way to continue to enjoy his lifelong passion. Ed also is a staunch Cubs fan. Because he has a very brief attention span, Ed is not able to participate in either activity, but he enjoys when a staff person reads highlights of the game from the daily newspaper and jokes with him about his Cubs hat.

## Interpersonal Approaches within Clusters

Just as the activities must be carefully adapted to match the functional ability of the person with dementia, the interpersonal approaches that are used to engage people in activities or an ADL must be carefully adapted and based on the core identity and the functional ability of each person. The approaches described by Taft et al. (1997), as well as approaches described by others (e.g., Bell & Troxel, 1997; Kitwood & Bredin, 1992), all have utility in promoting effective communication with people with dementia. However, they are not equally appropriate for each person with dementia or equally appropriate throughout a person's illness. Trial and error is one way of learning about the appropriateness of an approach; however, there are ways of selecting approaches that are less distressing for both the person with dementia and the person who cares for him or her. Interpersonal approaches are much more likely to be effective if matched to a person's core identity.

Startling a person with dementia, especially if approaching him or her from behind, is not likely to elicit a positive response. Bob, a nursing assistant, was having a congenial conversation with Alan, a resident with Alzheimer's disease, as they walked down a hall. As they passed through a doorway, Bob fell behind, and Alan focused on another staff person who addressed him as he and Bob entered the room. Bob lightly touched Alan on the back of his shoulder and said, "See you later." Alan turned and punched him. On reflection, Bob realized that this occurred because Alan was startled and felt the need to protect himself. Sheila always has been a bit of a practical joker. She delights in quietly approaching a staff member, standing behind him or her, and startling the person when he or she turns around. She also is delighted when this is done to her or especially when she catches someone in the attempt. The playfulness that brings such pleasure to Sheila would be totally inappropriate to use with Alan. Thus, selecting a playful approach, like selecting any other approach, must be based on knowledge of the person and his or her current functional ability.

Successful approaches most often are selected because of a fit with a person's sense of him- or herself and appropriateness in a specific situation. Often, the "how" and not the "what" is critically important. People with dementia can and do make allowances if they perceive that one's "heart is in the right place" and that one sincerely cares about them. A less-than-optimal approach may be successful if one is genuine and the person with dementia senses a true connection.

Subtlety in employing an approach or making an adaptation in an activity is essential. It is a conscious and purposeful effort to provide assistance in a way that is not obvious and that does not call attention to a particular difficulty or loss. It is using an approach or adaptation that enhances a person rather than one that merely avoids diminishing a person. For example, during a music group session, Marion got up and walked around the room, seemingly looking for something. In response to a staff member's offer of help, Marion replied, "I need to find the bathroom! How do I get out of this gracefully?" The staff person's response was, "Let's dance our way out." She and Marion danced out of the room and giggled about their unusual exit on the way to the bathroom. This approach changed the situation by lightening the mood, not simply avoiding embarrassment for Marion.

## What Clusters Are Not

Just as it is important to describe a process accurately, it is sometimes helpful to be clear about what a process is not. Clustering is matching all of the elements of the milieu as closely as possible to the abilities and needs of people with dementia. The purpose of clustering is not to group people by disease classifications, stages of a disease, or Mini-Mental State Examination scores. Given the heterogeneity of the symptoms of the disease, describing Alzheimer's disease in stages is a means of acknowledging the diversity of ability and need in a large population. However, the clinical experience of the authors has shown that stages are not necessarily descriptive of an individual's particular retained skills and needs. Clustering evolved out of millieu and practice that sought to provide the most comfortable milieu and activities that are appropriate for an individual's remaining abilities.

Clustering is based on the person's predominant characteristics and abilities, not on a single impairment. It is based on the totality of a person's characteristics, carefully balancing all of the person's strengths and abilities. Homogeneous clusters are not an attempt to create groups with *identical* characteristics but groups with *similar* characteristics. It is not about grouping people according to the lowest common denominator of functional ability. For instance, Ruth was asked to leave a previous adult day center because she was consistently incontinent. Ruth is a lady with great self-respect and social awareness. She is very alert in many ways, articulate, and aware of and responsive to others. Despite her incontinence, she is clustered with a group that is generally continent because the majority of her strengths are a fit with that group's skills.

Clustering does not just mean one group working on crafts while another is participating in a music activity. Most settings that provide services for older people offer diverse types of activities to accommodate a wide range of interests. However, this often means that the activities are designed to address interests, not differing abilities, which is the basis of clustering. Clustering assumes different strengths and abilities that require different adaptations to ensure success in the activity or task.

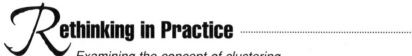

# $\mathcal{R}$ethinking in Practice

### Examining the concept of clustering

*Clustering is something we do naturally. We tend to associate with people who have similar interests and abilities. When we are in a group of people who have very different interests and abilities, we may feel uncomfortable and may have feelings of incompetence, inadequacy, or boredom. We can analyze the cause of our feelings and do something to change the situation; however, most people with dementia cannot do the same. Think about how you feel when you are out of your element. What is your response? A study of people in nursing facilities found that one of the most consistently reported needs was "to continue being who I am" (Burger, Fraser, Hunt, & Frank, 1996). Ask yourself the following questions:*

Do the physical, social, and cultural environments in a care setting that you know achieve this need?

Do the people with dementia seem to be out of their element?

What is the response of people with dementia?

Does it differ appreciably from your response in a similar situation?

*Think about clustering. In what ways would this concept help people you know with dementia continue to be who they are?*

Facilitating the use of retained skills and abilities is critical to prevent excess disability, or more disability than can be accounted for by the disease process. Although loss of ability is inevitable because of the progression of the disease, loss of skills and abilities because of lack of use can be avoided if activities are designed to use retained skills. Although, in general, excess disability is thought of in terms of physical functioning, it is probably more important to consider the social excess disability that is the result of a milieu that does not emphasize validating interpersonal interactions. Clustering according to ability helps create a milieu that facilitates using all of a person's skills, including communication and interpersonal skills (see Figure 8-1).

## Basis for Clusters

| What it is | What it is not |
|---|---|
| • Based on a person's current functional abilities<br>• Changes as people's abilities and program change<br>• Creating a homogeneous group<br>• Based on the majority of common functional characteristics | • Based on a person's interests (past or present)<br>• Static<br>• Creating an identical group<br>• Based on lowest common denominator of functional ability or most predominant "problem" behavior |

## Activities within a Homogeneous Cluster

| What they are | What they are not |
|---|---|
| • Focus on process<br>• Based on current interest and adapted to current functional level<br>• May be individual activities within a homogeneous cluster | • Focus on product<br>• Based on interest, but not adapted to current functioning<br>• Always involve a single activity in a group |

## Approaches within a Homogeneous Cluster

| What they are | What they are not |
|---|---|
| • Determined by person's core identity<br>• Adapted to fit person's current functional ability<br>• Develops relationships<br>• Encourages individual interactions | • Determined by random trial and error<br>• Static<br>• Focuses on "basic" care<br>• Implements rote techniques |

Figure 8-1.  Critical components of clustering.

# RECOGNIZING THE INDIVIDUAL CHARACTERISTICS OF PEOPLE WITH DEMENTIA

A person's ability to participate in an activity, complete a task, or interact with others is affected both by the impairment caused by Alzheimer's disease or a related dementia and by the environment of care, both physical and human. The authors' clinical experience has shown that people need very specific environmental supports, both physical and human, to facilitate the use of specific abilities and to meet specific needs. Therefore, the specific characteristics of the people in a group care setting must be carefully assessed to determine what accommodations need to be made to support the specific strengths of each person.

Assessing abilities and needs is based on the staff's clinical evaluation of people's abilities and needs rather than on formal testing. This practice was developed because methods that were commonly used to assess physical and cognitive function did not adequately measure the intangibles or subtleties (e.g., the essence of the person) that determine a person's ability. Research findings of significant differences in functional abilities of people clustered into groups validated the appropriateness of using clinical judgment to assess an individual's abilities and needs (Taft, Seman, Stansell, & Farran, 1992).

Assessing the characteristics of a person with dementia is not an event that occurs only on admission to a program. Assessment is a fluid, ongoing process that begins at admission. The purpose is to get to know the person as fully and completely as possible, not merely to list his or her care needs or life interests. This assessment is accomplished through a variety of means, such as conversations with the person with dementia, family members, and others who care for the person and observations of the response of the person to a setting or activity. Although assessing a person is certainly enhanced by talking with family and others who have known the person over time, this is not the only means of learning about the essence or core identity of the person.

Knowing occurs in many ways. Over the years, people with dementia and people caring for them have shared their knowledge. Some of what the authors have learned about excellence in observation and understanding the meaning of nonverbal behaviors was taught to them by Dorothy Smith, a program assistant who had little formal education but did have great wisdom and understanding of others. From her they learned the importance of careful and caring observation, that is, really seeing and being attentive to a person. She taught them much about the caring ways of knowing a person. For example, it is in the small moments of day-to-day interactions that people reveal their essential self or character. By learning to observe people with care, one can learn to distill or extract the meaning that a particular behavior may have. This is more than a quick impression based on a person's body language in a given circumstance; it is a process of coming to know a person through time. For instance, it is knowing that when Teddy pulls up his pants leg, he needs to use the bathroom. Sharing observations and impressions with others who also have direct and intimate contact with the person with dementia facilitates the process of piecing together a coherent understanding of him or her.

The purpose of the assessment process is to determine both the person's abilities and disabilities. Traditionally, health care assessments were problem focused to determine the specific problems requiring assistance or treatment. In acute health care settings attention is in general focused on providing the care needed to resolve a specific problem. This model is probably best described by nursing theorist Dorothy Orem (1980). In this theory of self-care, healthy adults are able to initiate and perform their own self-care. The role of the nurse is to provide only as much assistance as is needed to help the person return to a state of self-care. The nursing role may be wholly compensatory (i.e., the patient has no role in care), supportive/educative (i.e., patient is responsible for care/nurse provides education), or partly compensatory (i.e., the patient and the nurse perform care together). In this context it is easy to understand the problem focus of nursing assessment. In dementia care settings the role of the person providing care is to mitigate the impact of the disease on the person by supporting the person and his or her strengths while compensating for his or her losses. Therefore, the assessment focuses on the whole person and the context of that person's life. The following sections look at areas to consider in assessment by using one person, Marion, as an example.

## Core Identity

Probably the most important and most elusive component of the assessment is learning about the person's core identity or essence: who he or she is and what he or she values. This knowledge is important because it is helpful to understand the person's concept of self and lifelong coping style. For example, was the person characteristically stubborn, hard working, or lighthearted? Through time, how the person expresses him- or herself may change, but the essence of the person seems to remain stable. Knowledge of a person's core identity is one of the essential intangibles when planning activities that are appropriate for the person or when selecting an approach to care. Marion was a person with a strong sense of self and deep concern for others, especially children and people she referred to as "the less fortunate." She was a person with great perseverance, a sense of propriety, and a sense of humor, including the ability to laugh at herself. She also was a person with real strength of character and, although tactful, was not afraid to tell someone what she thought.

## Social History

To help answer the question "Who is this person?" we need to know how this person has lived his or her life (e.g., family; children; education; work; social, religious, military, and volunteer activities). The emphasis is on the meaning these things have to the person. For example, was work a way to support the family, or did it have another meaning? What relationships were especially important or difficult? It also is helpful to learn the stories of a person's life that have become family legends, such as the time Mom set the kitchen on fire because she was finishing a Halloween costume while fixing dinner. Marion came from a large and close family and grew up in a small midwestern town. She went to Catholic school, got married after her second year of college, and raised three daughters. When the girls were small, she was an active volunteer in the community and at the church and school they attended. The church always was an important part of her life. When her husband died at age 45, Marion went to work for the American Red Cross. She was director of the local chapter for many years. She saw her work as a continuation of her volunteer work, and in addition to being a way to support herself, it was a way to help others. When she could no longer live alone, her daughters moved her to a "senior apartment complex" in the city where they live. When she needed more assistance, her daughters bought a two-story apartment building, and they all moved in together. Marion enjoyed being with her daughters, and as a protective mother, she was concerned about their well-being.

## Life Interest

Although it is important to learn about a person's interests throughout his or her life, these interests are more than a list of hobbies and activities. Marion was a "people person," and she was not highly skilled at traditional homemaking tasks; cooking and sewing were necessary tasks, not points of pride. She played bridge in a club that was serious about cards—bridge was her passion. She never was interested in sports of any kind; her only outdoor activity was gardening. She used to really enjoy reading but no longer reads the daily newspaper. She loved music, especially show tunes.

## Communication

Communication impairments are a symptom of dementia that must be explored; thus, it is important to learn about a person's word-finding difficulties, ability to express needs and wants, and so forth. It is also important to learn about the person's method of response to these difficulties. Does he or she become frustrated or angry, ask for help, abandon the effort, or laugh about it? We must learn about the person's lifelong patterns of expressing him- or herself. For example, was he or she a person who expressed her feelings openly or did she keep them to him- or herself? Marion was an incredibly articulate person, with only a few remaining word-finding skills on admission to an adult day program. Her response to her word-finding difficulties often was, "Isn't this crazy? I know that I know that word." When the word was supplied to her, she would laugh and say, "Yes, that's it! Isn't this a silly thing?" The impressive social skills, communication patterns, and nonverbal communication skills that she had honed throughout her lifetime of interacting with others in a straightforward and sensitive way were evident, even when she could no longer use words coherently.

## Ways of Relating to Others

Like many characteristics, how a person relates to others is often a lifelong pattern that is retained throughout a dementing illness. How important have social relationships been to this person through life? Was this person more comfortable at home with family? Did this person enjoy being part of a group of people? How did this person relate to others in the family or to friends? How does the person relate to others now? Is the person comfortable with physical contact? Marion was an affectionate person, with an ability to, as one of her daughters put it, "give hugs at just the right time." She was a very responsible person, always taking care of everybody. She was close to her family and had a close-knit group of friends. Throughout her illness, Marion was an affectionate, social person who continued to express concern for others. "We can get it done if we all work together" was a phrase she used frequently.

## Cognitive Status/Judgment

Although cognitive testing is an important component of a diagnostic workup, it is not the kind of assessment that is recommended to determine how to best provide care. This testing is informative but does not provide real direction in care provision. Is this person aware of his or her illness? What is the person's response? What is the person's general level of understanding of the world around him or her? Does the person recognize and know how to use a spoon? What kinds of cues are helpful to him or her? Marion was aware of her illness but was not about to be defined by it. On admission to the program, she was alert and fairly independent, only needing a few wayfinding cues to help her get to the bathroom on time. Marion's judgment and cognitive capacity diminished as the disease progressed, but her conviction and courage did not.

## Responsiveness to the Environment

People with dementia vary considerably in their capacity to cope with the impact of the sensory stimulation in the environment. How does the physical environment affect this person? Is the person easily distracted? Is the person troubled by or curious about sounds in the environment? Marion was easily distracted but also easily redirected to an activity or a task. When she was admitted to the adult day program, she could focus on an activity for 15 to 20 minutes. As the disease progressed, she could only focus for 2 to 5 minutes, but she continued to respond with warmth and curiosity to people and things in the environment.

## Physical Functional Capacity

In assessing a person's capacity for physical functioning, it is critical to assess the functional skills that can be used within the context of a prosthetic environment. This assessment of function does not determine the extent of loss of independent functional ability. It is like assessing the ability of a person with an above-the-knee amputation to walk with a prosthesis—that is, is the person able to manage on an uneven surface, on a slippery sidewalk, and so forth? The following lists items that should be noted in an assessment of function (the list is supplemented by examples from Marion's assessment):

- Sensory changes—Deficits such as hearing, vision, and so forth; Marion wore thick glasses and was nearly blind when she misplaced them.
- Motor coordination—Motor planning deficits or coordination problems; Marion had considerable difficulty with eye–hand coordination and usually needed help with buttons and zippers. Marion's apraxia became quite severe, and she needed help with all activities requiring coordination, such as dressing or sitting in a chair.
- ADLs—Assistance that would be needed to help this person function as independently as possible (e.g., eating, toileting, grooming); on admission to the facility, Marion could eat without assistance, if her meat was precut and the correct utensils were supplied one at a time. She needed to be reminded to go to the bathroom, but once there, she could perform all of the necessary tasks independently because she only wore pants with an elastic waist. As the dementia progressed, she became much less independent and more apraxic. She needed assistance with all ADLs.

## Health

It is important to know the person's health history as well as current health status and medications. It is especially crucial that the assessment cover self-care deficits. Marion had been a very healthy person throughout her life. Just before admission to the facility, a mild diabetic condition had been diagnosed, which could be controlled by diet. However, she could not remember that she was diabetic and needed to be reminded that she should not eat cookies (a lifelong passion).

The skill that is involved in providing care for Marion and others lies in our ability to learn the important background information about the person and then integrate it with the person's present capacity. It is possible to provide minimally adequate care with a one-size-fits-all approach. However, by knowing a person's unique needs and abilities, we can enable him or her to experience continuity rather than loss as he or she goes about daily life.

## CLUSTERING INDIVIDUALS INTO GROUPS BASED ON FUNCTIONAL ABILITIES

Successfully engaging people with dementia in a group setting is enhanced by clustering people into groups with others of similar skills and abilities and by developing activities that use the strengths and skills of the group members. The characteristics of the people in a group care setting and the characteristics of the physical and human environments determine the number of groups that are needed and can be accommodated.

As one considers clustering people into groups with others of similar skills and needs, one should consider all of the characteristics of each person in a group setting. However, because activities must be strengths-based, it is imperative that each person's strengths be considered carefully. Identifying and supporting the person's strengths is the staff members' primary concern. To facilitate the use of these strengths and retained skills, staff members need to compensate for disease-related losses and mitigate the impact of those losses on the person's functional ability.

Although each person possesses unique individual characteristics, there are some commonalties in function and in groups that experienced clinicians have observed in a variety of group care settings. As the characteristics of people in a specific setting are examined, the following examples of possible clusters may be helpful. The characteristics described are only quick thumbnail sketches, not comprehensive descriptions of characteristics of people who may be clustered within a group.

## Sample Cluster A

Sample Cluster A consists of people who are able to communicate verbally and nonverbally, still have strong interpersonal skills, and in general display socially appropriate behavior. Although their short-term memory is fairly impaired, these individuals develop a general familiarity with routines and have sufficient attention span to participate in discussion or reminiscence activities for at least 20–30 minutes with minimal refocusing. Although they continue to be mostly independent in ADLs, these people need environmental cues to support independent functioning. If clustered into a group, friendships, a sense of group cohesiveness, and a familiarity with expectations often will develop. Transitions from one place to another or one activity to another cause minimal confusion, and these people exhibit minimal levels of anxiety.

## Sample Cluster B

The characteristics of people with very short attention spans are widely known in the field of dementia care. Sample Cluster B comprises people with an attention span of

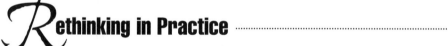

# *R*ethinking in Practice
### *Identifying the characteristics of people in a group setting*

*Because activity programming can be successful only if activities use a person's skills, clusters are based on remaining abilities as well as needs. The first step in clustering people according to ability is to identify the characteristics of people in a program. Consider the strengths, abilities, and needs of specific people in the following areas:*

Core identity
Attention span, ability to concentrate on
 a task
Level of attentiveness to others in the
 environment
Response to stimulation in the
 environment
Sensory capacity

Coping skills
Communication skills and styles
Physical functioning capacity
Cognitive capacity
Interests
Retained skills
Health

*Use one person as an example and spend time learning about and getting to know the person.*

2–5 minutes, who are highly distractible and mobile, and who have very poor short-term and highly impaired long-term memory and limited verbal communication skills. They are usually called "wanderers and pacers" or "rummagers and pillagers." In addition, they are often labeled "verbally abusive" or even "physically aggressive." These individuals also can be called spontaneous, curious, and highly social. They are comfortable expressing affection through touch and other nonverbal methods. Many share readily and adapt easily to most transitions. These characteristics can be accommodated in a group setting without medication or using physical restraints, if the milieu is carefully adapted to focus on the individuals' strengths. They are physically active, interact with people and objects in the environment, and are able to seek stimulating experiences.

## Sample Cluster C

Another group of people whose needs are widely known are those who have a lot of anxiety, are highly distractible, and have poor short-term memory and difficulty following a group discussion. Although they are social and more cognitively intact than those in Sample Cluster B, people in Sample Cluster C can refocus a group quickly. People can be fully engaged one minute, then a distraction occurs, such as a telephone ringing or a person entering or leaving the room, and the attention of the whole group is redirected. The potential of people in this sample cluster becomes quickly apparent when their strengths are considered. These are people who have high energy levels, the ability to communicate verbally and nonverbally, an awareness of changes in the environment, the ability to spontaneously interact with staff and other clients/residents, and the ability to manage anxiety if engaged in a task that focuses energy and attention and provides an outlet for physical energy. Often, they are fairly independent in ADLs but need some reminders and verbal cues.

## Sample Cluster D

Sample Cluster D is people who have profoundly impaired short-term memory, who are easily overstimulated, and who are overwhelmed by activity around them. These people seem startled by noise in the environment rather than curious about it. Many have very poor verbal skills, may retreat from a group (physically or emotionally), and may not be very physically active. Although these individuals have profound impairments, they still have strengths that can be used to engage them in activities that provide structure and stimulation without being overwhelming. They have the ability to interact verbally or nonverbally with others on a one-to-one basis or in a small group; may be able to participate in their ADLs with assistance (e.g., cues, special set-ups for lunch); and can complete familiar tasks such as folding, polishing silver, opening mail, or reading the newspaper.

There may be others in a setting who share many of the strengths and abilities of the people in Sample Cluster A but who need a hands-on component in an activity to maintain focus. Although these people seem to have relatively intact long-term memory, they have difficulty maintaining focus and concentration during an abstract discussion group. Others who share many characteristics of the people described in Sample Cluster D may be so sensitive to others in the environment that they may not be able to tolerate being in a group of more than four people. Being in a larger group or in a noisy environment may overwhelm them to the point that they may not even be able to eat or stand.

Many care environments have people with minimal impairments. Most of the skills that they have developed over a lifetime remain intact, and they may be very resistant to being taken care of. These people may have a need to discuss their experience with peers and also to continue their life patterns and interests. In most settings there will be people whose skills and needs are not easily categorized. It is for this reason that clusters are formed according to the preponderance of members' characteristics. It is also the reason for taking into account intangibles or those qualities about a person that are sometimes difficult to quantify but are such defining characteristics that the quality is apparent to everyone. Some people with especially strong social skills appear to have fewer impairments than they actually do. These people may test well and appear to be able to do things that are beyond their actual capacity. The best fit for a person may be determined by his or her comfort level as exhibited by the amount of participation in activities.

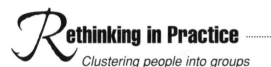

# $\mathcal{R}$ethinking in Practice

### Clustering people into groups

*Most of us gravitate toward other people with similar interests and abilities. This natural process of clustering provides each of us with the opportunity to focus on his or her abilities and relationships with those whom we find compatible. Clustering people with dementia into groups with others with similar skills and interests provides the same opportunities for developing peer relationships and focusing on abilities. It is imperative that clustering be based on the preponderance of commonalties in function and not simply on the person's most obvious problem in functioning.*

*Using the information from the assessment exercise (identifying the characteristics of people in a group setting), think about the following questions:*

What are some of the distinct differences among the people in the group?
In what ways are these differences communicated or revealed?
How do these differences make it difficult for each person to be comfortable and enjoy group activities?
What are some of the similarities in abilities and needs?

*Consider how many clusters are needed to provide an optimal environment for each person.*

Is this number realistic, considering the space and people available to provide care and lead activities? If not, what number of clusters can be accommodated?
Considering the commonalties among people, what clusters could be created to fit the available resources and still provide a comfortable milieu for each person?

# CREATING A MILIEU THAT IS SUPPORTIVE
# OF INDIVIDUAL CHARACTERISTICS OF PEOPLE IN EACH CLUSTER

People who have tried to develop an activity that they believe will get everyone in the unit involved know that this is truly an impossible mission. For instance, it is almost impossible to conduct a reminiscence group with people who are easily distracted in a room where a number of other things are happening. Neither a single activity nor a single activity space is universally effective for such a diverse group. For example, Brawley (1997) contended that one of the most innovative and positive changes in designing space for people with dementia has been the move from "one large communal activity space to a variety of smaller activity spaces" (p. 182). This change obviously requires a significant financial commitment from the leadership of an organization and an equally strong commitment from formal and informal leadership among the staff to design a program that effectively uses the resources that these spaces provide to benefit people with dementia. Clustering is a means of bringing all of the elements of the environment together—physical, social, and cultural—to support each person's abilities. Specific characteristics of each cluster provide direction for specific designs in the physical environment and for creation of a social environment that is supportive of the person and activities that use each person's skills.

Although multiple spaces that are designed specifically to support specific functional abilities are certainly the ideal, staff often use existing space that is less than ideal to cluster people into groups for activities based on the specific abilities of the people in the group. Space at the end of a hallway can be used for active games; space in the dining room can be used for many different kinds of activities. Activity space does not need to be single-use space (e.g., craft rooms, music rooms). It is probably more efficient to select a variety of spaces that are versatile and can be used in multiple ways.

The physical space must support function. A study carrel may help a person who is highly distractible to focus more effectively on an individual task than would space at a table with other people. A small room without distractions is a more effective space for a discussion group than is a large room. Some people may experience difficulty hearing in a large space. Others may be distracted in a space where there are several doors that are opened frequently or with people entering and leaving the room.

The following examples of clusters show ways to create a milieu that both supports the strengths of individual group members and accommodates their losses. These samples are intended to spark your thinking, not to provide rigid guidelines that must be followed. The samples are thumbnail sketches rather than an exhaustive discussion of all of the environmental components that are necessary to create a validating and stimulating milieu.

## Sample Cluster A

The primary requirement of the physical environment for people in Sample Cluster A is a space for activities that minimizes distractions (e.g., telephones ringing, overhead paging, people not involved in the group who are interrupting activities), compensates for losses (e.g., hearing, vision, wayfinding), and provides for safety needs. Given the strengths of this group, the role of staff is more of a facilitator or orchestrator than it is a group leader. People in this group can articulate their feelings and wishes fairly well, so the role of staff is to follow the lead of the group members in planning activities and offering choices of activities to be developed. In planning outings or special events it is especially important for staff to gather information about individual interests from group members. Due to their short-term memory losses, people with dementia may not remember making the plans, but their interests can be incorporated in the activity program. The kinds of activities and outings that are appropriate for people in Sample Cluster A are diverse and require staff who have the capacity to provide subtle supports to promote a sense of competence.

Staff must appreciate the many abilities of people in this group. These individuals often are very aware of the impact of their dementing disease on their functional capacity and are sensitive about being asked to participate in an activity that does not use their abilities fully. Most adults respond quite negatively to actual or perceived infantilization, and it can be a particularly sensitive issue for people in this group. In a discussion about this issue, Frank said, "You do, I mean, we do, need help from others. I guess we have to accept it and understand it has to be on someone else's time schedule, not yours . . . that's the hard part. It's also hard when you may not be ready for this or that help. Sometimes when you need some help, your kids think you need help with everything. People want to help so much they get in the way. They don't intend to, but you are made to feel like a baby or a fool that doesn't know any better."

Staff need to be sensitive and open to discussing the impact of Alzheimer's disease on a person's life and relationships or the concerns that a person may express about other family matters. These discussions often occur spontaneously when staff create a supportive social environment. During an exercise group, the topic of anger came up and Lorraine said, "My husband has what I do, Alzheimer's, but he's worse. I try to take care of myself and him. It's so hard and so sad. Sometimes I get so mad and angry. That's an easier way than feeling the hurt and not knowing what's next."

Staff must be alert to the needs of the people in the group. If alert and lively discussions are the norm, then staff need to be careful about the pacing of the activities and choices provided so that people do not feel undue pressure to perform or share. It is especially critical that staff be subtle about safety issues to avoid causing feelings of loss of control in people's lives. Subtle compensations for losses also are needed at mealtime. Although people in Sample Cluster A tend to be social, social interaction does not usually extend to meals because of the concentration that is needed to attend to the task at hand. Staff should respect this need for concentration and avoid unnecessary chatting and distraction.

Staff also should provide needed assistance with meals that does not call attention to a person's motor and coordination deficits. For example, Elaine is quite socially aware and articulate. She is embarrassed by her apraxia, which presents significant difficulties at mealtime. Finger foods were provided in a way that was respectful of Elaine and sensitive to her feelings. Staff said, "The cook knows you are not fond of stew and thought you might like to try some of the tea sandwiches she made. Any of you stew lovers want to try one?" This gave Elaine an opportunity to eat food that was manageable for her without calling attention to her deficit.

## Sample Cluster B

If individuals are clustered in a group and provided a physical environment with adequate space to walk and explore, things to investigate (e.g., props to discover and use, sometimes in very inventive ways, sometimes in very familiar ways), and positive interactions with other people, individuals who may exhibit behaviors that have been described as challenging are less difficult for the staff because the milieu has been designed to accommodate them (see Sample Cluster B on p. 126). Because people in Sample Cluster B tend to respond to visual stimulation, investigating or arranging items that have been provided for this purpose is more appropriately described as sorting rather than rummaging or pillaging. The person is not constantly receiving negative sanctions such as "Stop!" "Quit that!" "Put that back; it's not yours." A steady diet of negative sanctions would make anyone grumpy, not only people with dementia. ("Grumpy" is a word that we use to describe our own behavior; more often the person with dementia is described as "agitated" or even "violent.")

Staff-initiated activities are designed to accommodate the brief attention span of people in Sample Cluster B. Although there are numerous activities that these people can still be successful in doing, group activities must be created to fit the need to move to something else after a short interval and to return to the activity without disrupting others in the group. Because people in this sample cluster have the capacity to seek an activity that is of interest to them, much of their activity in a given day is self-initiated or subtly facilitated. When they are actively engaged in something of interest to them and are not being continuously redirected to an activity that is beyond their capacity, they experience less frustration and less agitation.

Because the individuals in this cluster are often "on the move," staff need to be especially attentive to safety issues such as watching for untied shoelaces, dropping finger foods designed to be eaten on the move (creating the possibility of slipping and falling), and exploring in areas that could present a danger. Given the energy used by people in this group, frequent snacks and drinks also are an important consideration.

## Sample Cluster C

A physical environment that reduces extraneous distractions is essential for older adults in Sample Cluster C. A space that is large enough to allow movement without being disruptive and to accommodate multiple activities simultaneously is needed. Study carrels, individual desks, a workbench, and multiple tables are necessary workspaces for people in this group. Activities need to focus on hands-on tasks rather than on something that is not physically involving, such as a discussion group.

Hands-on activities such as puzzles, painting, repairing a small appliance, or wood-working can be done individually in a group setting and provide opportunities for people to socialize without being disruptive. Activities such as folding clothes, napkins for lunch, or newsletters; watering the grass; or mowing the lawn also can provide the person with dementia the needed opportunity to make a contribution as well as enjoy an activity. Activities need to be geared to the skills developed over a lifetime to provide the most opportunity for success. Active games or music are often successful means of involving most of the people in a group activity.

Although fairly independent in ADLs, people in Sample Cluster C usually need reminders and verbal cues to be successful. People in the group also may need frequent reassurance and redirection to maintain their focus on an activity. Responses to concerns need to be timely and specific to older adults, such as, "Your son Tom is picking you up after he gets off work." Staff need to be alert to any changes in the milieu that could potentially increase the anxiety level of an individual or group and provide immediate reassurance about the change. When someone walks into a room,

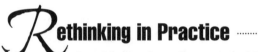

# *R*ethinking in Practice

### *Considering the milieu needed for each cluster*

*Milieu is critical to the successful functioning of each cluster. All of the components of the environment—physical, social, and cultural—must be thoughtfully assessed to create a milieu that is supportive of and responsive to each person within the group. After determining how many clusters can be accommodated, consideration of the following questions may help spark your thinking about necessary environmental supports.*

*Think about the physical space needed for each group.*

How do the people in each group use space?

What is the people's response to environmental stimuli, and what modifications in environmental stimuli need to be made to minimize distress and distraction?

What specific furniture or arrangements of furniture would facilitate optimal functioning for each person?

What supplies (e.g., activity, dietary) are needed for this group?

*Consider the different social supports needed for each group.*

How many staff persons are needed for the group to function smoothly?

What kinds of activities are most appropriate for this group?

What general adaptations are needed to ensure the success of an activity in this group?

*Consider the different ADL supports that are needed for each group.*

What changes in the physical environment are needed to facilitate serving meals in a specific group?

How many staff members are needed to assist this group at mealtime?

What adaptations or special setups are needed to facilitate eating with minimal personal assistance?

attention often is diverted from the activity or task at hand to questions about the new person: Why is she here? What does she want? A quick explanation such as, "Linda is bringing us some juice to have when we finish exercising," will answer the questions and diminish the anxiety that results from unanswered questions.

Staff also should pay attention to the rhythm and pace of activities. Hall and Buckwalter's (1987) model responding to diminishing stress thresholds, although important in any dementia care setting, is critical for the people in this group. Because people in this cluster have little capacity to modulate any stress or anxiety by themselves, their levels of anxiety can escalate dramatically. It becomes the staff's responsibility to compensate for this deficit by alternating the kinds of activities that are provided. Quieter and individually focused activities such as art are alternated with more active group games such as balloon volleyball.

Staff also need to be aware of compatibility issues among the members of this group. Misperceptions and misunderstandings in social interactions are common as language skills become further impaired. Often, these misunderstandings can be avoided by planned seating during an activity or can be short-circuited by reframing comments. Most of the members of this group need assistance with wayfinding; those who can still use the bathroom independently need help finding their way back to the group. If the group leader leaves the group to help them, then the whole group will lose focus. Therefore, it is important to have "float" staff available to help with redirection or to lend a hand where needed.

## Sample Cluster D

People in Sample Cluster D have lost the ability to filter out extraneous noises and activity, so that must be done for them. Means of reducing environmental distractions include no overhead paging, not playing background music, and using nonverbal cues rather than talking. Rooms that are designed to be visually interesting without being overstimulating seem to be most appropriate for this group's comfort level. Activities are most often based on sensory rather than verbal modalities. Staff need to pace the activities so that people in this group are not overwhelmed and can participate in the activity. Staff also need to provide familiar activities and opportunities for satisfying interactions with others, for example, seating a person next to someone who is compatible. This milieu requires supportive staff who communicate support and validation verbally and nonverbally.

## PUTTING IT ALL TOGETHER AND MAKING IT WORK

Rita Mae Brown (1984) defined insanity as "doing the same thing over and over again, but expecting a different result each time." Some of us who are particularly persistent make ourselves and those around us even crazier by not merely trying the same thing over and over but by putting more and more energy into what is not working (or doing more and more of what is not working). Because people with dementia cannot easily adapt to the structure of existing programs due to the impairment resulting from the disease, we need to stop focusing on what is not working well and try a different approach.

Programs need to be designed to organize care that is good for both staff and people with dementia. Clustering evolved from clinical experience and a concerted effort to create a program that works for everyone. By clustering people with similar skills and needs into groups, people are more comfortable and able to use their retained skills. There is less frustration because they are not being asked to do things that are beyond or beneath their individual capacity. In addition, staff feel more comfortable because the activities are more successful. There is less frustration and fewer feelings of inadequacy and more time and energy to connect with each person and relate in ways that are validating, both for the person with dementia and for the staff. Everyone has been set up to succeed rather than fail.

By now you may be saying to yourself, "Yes, this makes sense . . . this really fits my personal experience, but what can I do?" or, "I'm only one person, and at my workplace, we really can't do this because we don't have _____ (insert reason)." Admittedly what is being advocated is somewhat revolutionary in the way we think about people with dementia as well as the way care is provided. However, to paraphrase Maya Angelou, every revolution starts with a single person, and this revolution is way beyond the single-person phase. There are many people who firmly believe that people with dementia retain their humanity and many life skills despite their losses throughout the course of the illness. There are many people who firmly believe that we can and must make changes in the way that we care for people with dementia. You are not a solitary person but are one of a growing number of people who are passionately committed to providing care for people with dementia in ways that recognize their humanity, abilities, and needs.

## REFERENCES

Bell, V., & Troxel, D. (1997). *The best friends approach to Alzheimer's care.* Baltimore: Health Professions Press.

Brawley, E.C. (1997). *Designing for Alzheimer's disease: Strategies for creating better care environments.* New York: John Wiley & Sons.

Brown, R.M. (1984). *Sudden death* (p. 68). New York: Bantam Books.

Burger, S., Fraser, V., Hunt, S., & Frank, B. (1996). *Nursing homes: Getting better care there.* San Luis Obispo, CA: American Source Books.

Hall, G.R., & Buckwalter, K.C. (1987). Progressively lowered stress threshold: A conceptual model for care of adults with Alzheimer's disease. *Archives of Psychiatric Nursing, 1*(6), 399–406.

Kitwood, T., & Bredin, K. (1992). Towards a theory of dementia care: Personhood and well being. *Ageing and Society, 12*, 269–287.

Neugarten, B. (1988). Personality and psychosocial patterns of aging. In M. Bergener, M. Ermini, & H.B. Stahelin (Eds.), *Crossroads in aging* (pp. 205–219). New York: Academic Press.

Orem, D. (1980). *Nursing: Concepts of practice.* New York: McGraw-Hill.

Silcox, S., & Cohen, P. (1987). *Adapting the adult day care environment for the demented older adult.* Springfield: Illinois Department on Aging.

Taft, L., Seman, D., Stansell, J., & Farran, C. (1992, September/October). Behavioral dimensions of dementia: A comparison of three program groups in adult day care. *American Journal of Alzheimer's Care and Related Disorders & Research,* 32–39.

Taft, L.B., Fazio, S., Seman, D., & Stansell, J. (1997). A psychosocial model of dementia care: Theoretical and empirical support. *Archives of Psychiatric Nursing, 11*(1), 13–20.

Ziggy. (n.d.). Available: http://www.quoteland.com/quotes/search/search.cgi?

# Reexamining Ways of Working with Families

*Traveler, there is no path; paths are made by walking.*

*Henry A. Kissinger*

Families are as different as are the individuals who are part of them. However, the way information, support, and guidance often are provided is not personal or individual. Many times, families are communicated to in a rote or "one-size-fits-all" manner. The approach can be very prescriptive in nature and representative of a narrow and at times inaccurate view of the disease process, care options, and support systems. Without a specific road map to follow, families often are left to find their own way, guided by misinformation and limited views.

Finding their own way would not necessarily be bad if families were equipped with accurate information and a more encompassing view of the disease process and care options, and if families were supported by care providers in a manner that is appropriate to their needs. Then, the decisions they make could be based on a more balanced view of what lies ahead, and the guidance given could be more specific to their individual and collective strengths and needs. To give this guidance, care providers must have a good understanding of how systems function and what families know about the disease and care and the possibilities that can emerge when the full picture is considered. By working with families individually, providers can educate and support them, explore possibilities, and find solutions that are right for them—creating a true family-centered partnership.

## UNDERSTANDING FAMILY SYSTEMS

A basic concept of family therapy theory is that families are systems whose members have interconnected and interdependent relationships and strive to maintain equilibrium or balance in the system (Foley, 1974). It is within the context of these relationships that each family member attempts to get his or her personal needs met, including emotional needs such as intimacy, self-expression, and purpose in life.

These concepts can help clinicians more clearly understand the impact that a family member with dementia has on the whole family system. Relationships within family systems are never static but change and evolve through the life cycle of a family in response to many events, including life transitions (e.g., having children, an ongoing illness). Family members continue to strive to get their personal needs met in the context of the changing family relationships while maintaining a balance within the system.

Families often are called "the true victim" because the person diagnosed with dementia is thought to be unaware of and untroubled by the disease. From a systems perspective, this view of the person with dementia leads to his or her being isolated from the rest of the family. However, we have learned that many people with dementia are aware of the changes that they are experiencing. Often, they are able to express a range of thoughts and feelings about the illness and their care, if families and others are open to hearing them. Families may need some encouragement to overcome the abundant misinformation about people with dementia and to maintain their relationships with them through open, supportive communication.

Communication, a key factor in the maintenance of relationships and attainment of needs satisfaction within a family, usually is affected fairly early in a dementing illness. Research has shown that fewer than half of the family members of people with Alzheimer's disease reported changes in relationships as a direct result of changes in the communication ability of the person with dementia (Orange, 1991). Family members sometimes describe feelings of loneliness and loss, even early in the illness, because they cannot discuss issues or problems in their usual manner. Families that are able to maintain supportive, satisfying relationships despite the changes caused by the illness seem to describe the caregiving experience positively. This is especially important because sustaining meaningful relationships is essential in helping the person with dementia support his or her identity and importance within the family.

Also important is to recognize that no two families are alike and that there is great diversity in family dynamics. Clinicians need to be sensitive to and respect differing cultural and/or religious beliefs that serve as the basis for a family's functioning. It is important that clinicians have a basic understanding of how a family functions and recognize especially supportive or difficult relationships and how these have been affected by the illness. They must understand that family members can still attain satisfaction of needs despite the changes in relationships.

## ADDRESSING THE IMPACT OF ONGOING ILLNESS ON FAMILY FUNCTIONING AND COPING ABILITY

The life cycle of a family does not stop when a family member is diagnosed with probable Alzheimer's disease. A family's response to the challenges of the illness is not only affected by family beliefs and patterns of functioning but also by other occurrences within the family system. Rolland (1994) contended that it is important to understand the impact of any ongoing illness on family functioning, in terms both of providing care needed by the individual family member and meeting the ongoing developmental needs of the family as a whole. Most families come together in times of an acute illness to focus on the care needs of the family member. Most families are able to incorporate the many competing needs of all family members, and meeting the ongoing needs of the person with dementia becomes a typical part of family functioning.

Clinicians should monitor the family's focus on caregiving needs, especially in times of transition in the family's life cycle or developmental phases, such as young adult children leaving home and starting their own families or older adult children retiring. Caregiving can overwhelm the family's resources, especially during traditional times of transition, resulting in dysfunction. These developmental phases or times of transition can be prolonged, or families can "get stuck" in a phase (Rolland, 1994). Families with relationship difficulties before onset of an illness may not be able to separate the person from the illness, or they may become so focused on providing care that other family needs cannot be met. Addressing all of the needs of these families may be beyond the resources of staff members who are providing care for people with dementia and may require referral to medical family therapists (see next section).

Many families are able to coordinate the care needed for the long term for a family member with dementia without major disruption in the developmental needs of other family members. For example, the teenage children in a family can alternate spending time after school with their grandmother with dementia, depending on their extracurricular activities. This arrangement not only meets the grandmother's care needs but also enriches the relationship between the children and their grandmother and enables the children to make a meaningful contribution to the family.

The first step in helping the individuals within a family system is to understand the emotional climate of a family and how it influences relationships. Bowen (1971) advocated genograms as a means of concisely and graphically describing a family system. Genograms can be a quick and nonthreatening way to elicit helpful information. For example, when asking about the family history of a person with dementia, we may learn that the person had taken care of her mother through a long illness. Often, if we are listening with empathy, not just asking questions and completing a form, family members feel comfortable expressing their own feelings. Comments such as, "In our family we take care of each other," or, "I am just not as strong as she was; I am not able to do that," provide critical information and understanding of family dynamics, capacities, and needs.

## IDENTIFYING THE STRENGTHS AND NEEDS OF EACH FAMILY

The relatively new field of medical family therapy provides direction for clinicians who are helping individuals and families to cope with health problems and ongoing illnesses, such as Alzheimer's disease. The two primary goals of this effort are to foster relationships within the family system so that the families can cope with a family member's illness and to promote a sense of autonomy and control in navigating the health care system (McDaniel, Hepworth, & Doherty, 1992). Although it is important to help families understand the biological impact of dementia, it is equally important not to medicalize every behavior of a person with dementia or attribute

# *R*ethinking in Practice

### *Using a genogram to help understand family systems*

*Because each family system has its own unique characteristics, beliefs, power structures, learning styles, and ways of solving problems to maintain balance within the system, it is critical to understand the dynamics of the family system and the beliefs that are the basis for the characteristics of the system. Consider the following genogram as an example. Then, make a genogram to describe a family you know, noting such characteristics as special relationships, problems, and strengths.*

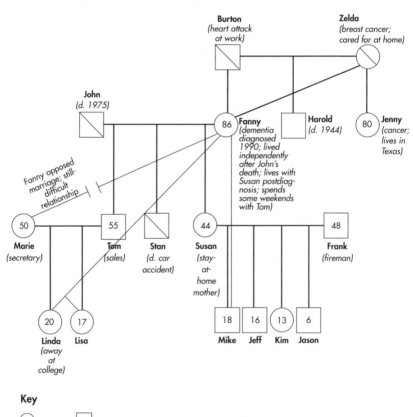

each behavior to a neurological impairment. It is important to ask family members whether a behavior, such as being stubborn or uncooperative, is a lifelong characteristic or a new behavior. If it is a new behavior, a change in the caregiving approach may result in a change in the behavior. If it is a lifelong characteristic, the behavior should not be viewed as a medical problem or symptom to be treated. Instead, we need to explore how this behavior has been accommodated within the family system and whether this approach will continue to work.

As family members describe the person and relationships within the family, it is important to identify the strengths and limitations of the person with dementia and his or her family. After identifying family characteristics, ways of coping, and needs, we can help them create plans to meet the challenges they are experiencing based on the strengths of the family. Encouraging open communication about both the biological component of the illness and the experience of the illness from

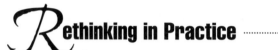

# *R*ethinking in Practice

*Exploring families' perceptions of illness and care*

*Families expect health care providers to ask questions and be prepared to answer questions about the illness and problems that the families are experiencing. By eliciting the family's perceptions of the illness and relationships, we also can discover much about the family's strengths, beliefs about the illness, and ways of coping and determine the assistance that they might need.*

*Review the following questions and compare them with questions asked at the time of admission to your setting:*

When did you first notice a memory problem?
What kinds of things seemed different?
What was your family member's response to these changes? What was your response?
How do memory problems affect your family member's functioning now?
What has been most problematic for him or her? For you? What has helped with these problems?
What do you fear most about dementia? What do you think will be the biggest struggle for you?
Has anyone else in your family experienced something similar? If so, how was care provided for him or her?
Where and with whom does your family member live now? How is this working out?
How much do friends and family help? Who and how much?
In what ways has this illness changed your daily life?
Have there been any recent changes in the family? Are any changes anticipated? What changes do you think will be needed as the disease progresses?
Have you thought about and talked with your family regarding plans for the long term?

*These questions and others like them provide information that help not only to understand the family but also to provide direction about the kinds of assistance that may be needed by and acceptable to the family.*

the perspective of the person with dementia and the family is important; however, clinicians must be sensitive to a family's communication styles. Many families exhibit great diversity in the way that feelings are discussed or expressed. Because the focus is on meeting the needs of the person with dementia and his or her family, it is imperative to be aware of this diversity and provide support to those involved. Many staff members fall into the habit of collecting information using a singular, generic approach of sitting across a table and filling out the forms in a rather systematic, chronological order. It is useful to think about approaching families and this important task individually, much as we try to individualize our approach to the person with dementia. By adapting our approach to accommodate a family's comfort level, these interactions often are far more productive.

For example, if a family member comes to a care setting filled with anxiety, it may be much kinder and far more useful to ask him or her to tell us what we could do to help. It is important to find out what kinds of questions we can answer or what concerns are most pressing. It often helps in establishing trust and rapport. Helping people with dementia and their families to feel a sense of control in dealing not only with the illness but also with the health care system is a critical role for all clinicians. Some families may only need factual information; other families may need a significant amount of education, support, and encouragement to feel competent in making decisions and taking on the role of advocate for the person with dementia.

## KEEPING REALISTIC EXPECTATIONS IN WORKING WITH FAMILIES

In addition to understanding the family as a system and the dynamics that contribute to a family's style of functioning and coping, it is important to focus on the primary responsibility of staff and the capacities and limitations of the care setting. For most clinicians, providing care for the person with dementia is the primary responsibility; thus, work with families probably is limited to helping them cope with the illness while maintaining a relationship with the person with dementia. This work can sometimes stretch families' available resources. Families who need more assistance than can be provided within the scope of the care setting should be referred to a family therapist or others who can help them work through issues that are outside the capacity of the care setting. Although some families can incorporate care for their relatives with dementia with minimal support, others may need a variety of support options to help minimize the stresses caused by the challenges of the illness. An objective third party, such as an eldercare attorney or a case manager, may be needed to help families arrange or coordinate care and services.

Use of a third party is especially important when working with complex family systems with multiple health or other family issues or legal problems that involve numerous health, social, and legal services. In these circumstances it is generally most helpful to identify the person in the family and/or in another agency who is coordinating the care of the person with dementia and deal directly and exclusively with that person. Having multiple contacts in these circumstances almost always leads to confusion and further difficulty for everyone involved.

Not only is it critical for clinicians and staff in care settings to maintain realistic expectations about their role in working with families but it is equally critical to understand families' expectations of them. Efforts to establish a foundation regarding expectations and overarching values, both the setting's and the family's, form a sound basis for a working relationship. If there are differences between the family's expectations and the capacities and limitations of the care setting, these need to be identified, discussed, and resolved to avoid problems in the relationship with the family. With the explosion of the numbers and types of resources and the rapid pace of health care decisions to be made, some vulnerable families may present themselves in a high state of anxiety or with an urgent need. Although it may be tempting for staff in a care setting to "close the deal" quickly, it serves no one's needs in the long run if the care setting is not the best fit for the person with dementia. This effort to refer to the setting that is the best fit and not merely adequate often

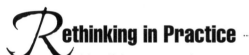

## ethinking in Practice

### Identifying expectations to meet needs

*It is important to identify as clearly as possible the strengths and needs of the person with dementia as well as of the family as a whole. Then it can be determined which needs can be met within the resources of the care setting and which needs require a referral to other resources. Consider the following questions:*

What educational needs do family members have? What educational needs do they identify? Can these needs be met in this setting or is another agency or resource more appropriate?

What needs for support are identified by the family? Does this needs identification appear to be realistic? Can these needs be met within the resources of the care setting?

What needs of the family are beyond the scope of the care setting?

*Many of the difficulties between families and clinicians in care settings can be attributed to differing expectations. These difficulties can be avoided by reaching an understanding about expectations early in the relationship. Families must be provided with information about the capacities and limitations of the care setting. Because families may be anxious at the time of the first meeting or on their loved one's admission to a care facility, it is important not only to have discussion but also to provide written information and to encourage ongoing discussion about questions or concerns. Ask questions to identify family expectations of the care setting, such as the following:*

What does the family expect of us?

Does the family understand what we can and cannot do?

How does the family define quality of life for the person with dementia?

Does this definition differ from the care setting's philosophy and practice? In what ways?

*These questions and others like them can help staff to more clearly understand when there is a good fit between the expectations of the family and the care setting. They also can point to areas that need to be negotiated, clarified, or referred to a more appropriate resource.*

will pay dividends later, in terms of goodwill from family members and the support of collegial relationships with other care settings in the community.

## ESTABLISHING OPPORTUNITIES FOR FAMILY-CENTERED PARTNERSHIPS

In many care settings, families have been treated as if their sole purpose were to provide medical history and demographic information on a "patient" (their family member) who could not self-report accurately. Beyond that, the role of family often was relegated to consenting to a procedure when the person was not capable of doing so or receiving a call about an accident or injury in which their family member was involved. This kind of communication cannot be construed as a relationship or partnership in any sense of the word. In many settings staff members may think of family members variously as visitors to be tolerated, interlopers, inconvenient, or nuisances. However, on days when the program or unit is short staffed or if the person has many needs, staff may seek out or readily accept family members as volunteer help. Only a few situations in health care settings exist in which the family is seen as the unit of care or as an integral and vital part of care, for example, in pediatrics or mental health family counseling.

Not all families want a partnership role with staff; others may want an active and involved role in planning and implementing care. While acknowledging that there are many kinds of partnerships between family members and staff that work well, some initial difficulties in transition need to be addressed. Families often are uncertain and uneasy about their ambiguous new role, once their relative begins to receive care outside the family unit. Some families may have trouble relinquishing control because they believe that no one could do as good a job providing care as they have done. Others may have provided care for so long that they have lost their identity or any structure to their life. They may have difficulty giving up the work that has defined their life for so long. Some families may be uncertain about how to help their relative obtain the best possible care when they no longer provide the majority of direct hands-on care themselves. Still other families may feel that they are just being tolerated or not included when their role is more ritualized or confined to the schedule imposed by the care setting, rather than in accordance with their needs and wishes. As with any change or transition, people need time to become accustomed to their new roles.

Some staff members believe that there is room for improvement in the quality of working relationships between them and involved family members. The challenges of long-term care invite and require that staff think about families differently. Many care environments have found opportunities to engage families in ways that are mutually satisfying (e.g., assistance with meals, personal care, activities) and, most important, that can achieve much better care for the person with Alzheimer's disease. To accomplish this transition to a successful partnership, we need to reevaluate our way of thinking and approaching care and to acknowledge the right of each family to define the kind of relationship that they want to establish. In health care systems of all kinds it is expected that staff members design and provide an individualized plan of care for each person in their care. Unfortunately, this concept has not consistently extended to our thinking about individualizing our approach to family members and the family unit as a whole.

In most care environments families continue to express varying degrees of interest and skill in providing care, yet we tend to take a singular approach to family work. We do not yet have a common language for describing these subtypes of family groups that have important implications for how we establish initial and ongoing contact. Perhaps we have many unspoken expectations about how we think that families should feel and behave and how they should relate to or care for their relative. It is likely that many of us think and feel the way we do about the family's role because of our own unique family experience. We must work so as not to impose that unconscious template of expectations on other individuals and their fami-

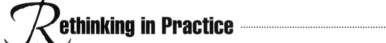

# *R*ethinking in Practice

*Exploring personal beliefs about family responsibility and illness*

*As a way of identifying our own deeply embedded values and expectations of families, it may be helpful to discuss these issues directly among staff. Because our individual views have such power to influence our clinical practice with families, it is critical that we be aware of these views and guard against imposing them on the families with whom we work. Our role is to assist families to clarify the values that are held most dear by their relative with dementia and to enable them to provide directly or to obtain the kind of care that is consistent with those ideals. Ask yourself the following questions:*

What do I personally believe is the responsibility of family members for one another?
How did I develop these values?
How have these values changed over time?
Do I feel free to do what I think is fair and reasonable for relatives in need, or do I defer to what others expect of me?
What feelings are brought forth in me when family members do not provide the kind of care for their relative with Alzheimer's disease that I think is right?
Do I truly respect the right of each family member to care for his or her relative in his or her own unique way?
To what extent am I able to set my value system aside and help families to be true to their wishes?
What family behaviors do I find most difficult to deal with?
What resources can I call on when I find that I need help maintaining my boundaries to enable families to make their own choices in care?
How would I feel if staff members in a health care setting judged my family or me based on their view of what our family should do?

*Developing sensitivity to our own values about families may facilitate communication and enable us to accept others' values.*

lies. If we are not conscious of our own biases, it is likely that families will sense our judgment of them in our tone and approach. This lack of acceptance of each family's uniqueness may erect barriers to ongoing communication.

The clinical literature offers limited guidance in identifying ways to distinguish the best clinical approach for working with various kinds of families who have a role in providing care for a family member with Alzheimer's disease. A common assumption and expectation of some staff members is that all families want to have a partnership with staff and that this goal is limited only by the lack of sufficient resources to do so. Many clinicians may assume that all families want the same detail and degree of information and involvement and that more is better. It is important to distinguish the needs of staff from those of families.

Many clinicians may feel a sense of personal and professional gratification when the opportunity arises for an ongoing and rich dialogue with families, with exchanges that seem to be mutually validating and enriching. It is important to acknowledge, however, that although shared dialogue may be rewarding for some families, it is not universally so. Some families may prefer another kind of relationship, and our efforts to impose our expectations on them can cause discomfort and may be unworkable. Some staff members believe that these close working relationships are "the reason I went into (name the profession)." We must keep our focus, not on our own needs but on the needs of families, who are at the heart of family-centered Alzheimer's care. Our approach should be selected based on the needs and preferences of the family, as long as the person's basic needs for care, safety, and well-being are met.

The reasons that families may prefer a more peripheral role are numerous, and it is their right to take such a role. Sometimes the clinical history or our observations may provide necessary clues for our understanding. Such data may help us to realize that the emotional connections among family members may have been strained or broken beyond repair. Families may have experienced sexually or physically abusive relationships, abandonment, emotional unavailability, a parent's or spouse's hypercritical nature, infidelity, or so forth. The person with Alzheimer's disease may appear to be short-changed by family members, but his or her personal and family biography may hold many clues as to the quality of relationships before the diagnosis. Some family members may believe that the care and oversight they now provide is all they can or all they are willing to give. Others may find a deeper involvement too painful. Some families may hope for the opportunity to share some of this information and try to grow beyond it; others may consider this information as history, not to be revisited. Clinical staff should be alert to opportunities to invite but not force dialogue within these families.

Staff members may assume that families who have brought their relative to live in a structured care environment have given their relative over to someone else and are now "free of the burden." However, a number of families are eager to maintain intimate contact and seek details about their relative's care. They may even wish to continue to provide or direct the person's care, such as assisting with meals or helping to bathe their loved one. These families may want to be informed about what and how much their family member ate for breakfast, when they last had a bowel movement, what specific activities they participated in, or other such information. What this suggests is that an effective partnership rests on this mutual understanding and set of clear expectations and on honoring the preference of family members for the information they want and need. Clinical staff members need to tailor their approach for each family and provide neither too much nor too little information to meet each family's needs. Staff should make every effort to provide the opportunity for families to assist in direct care if they wish to do so. This approach may ease the transition to a congregate care setting for the person with Alzheimer's disease and his or her family, or it may be an ongoing activity that is gratifying to some family members.

## REINTRODUCING ALZHEIMER'S DISEASE TO FAMILIES

On initial contact with a family, a care provider in any care setting should attend to several key items. These include ensuring that a comprehensive diagnostic evaluation has been completed, ensuring that the family has sufficient information about the disease and its progression, and determining that the family has access to useful and complete information about all appropriate care options and knows how to use that information to make appropriate choices. When a family presents themselves at a care setting, many clinicians make automatic assumptions that the family has sufficient and accurate information about the disease, but some families have limited, incorrect, outdated, or exaggerated information about Alzheimer's disease. Sometimes this information has come from ill-informed health care providers, friends, neighbors, family members, or the media. It is critical that families have an accurate foundation on which to build or continue relationships with their relative and facility staff.

Some families may seek services if they believe that their relative has Alzheimer's disease because he or she has become increasingly confused. With the numerous stories about Alzheimer's disease in the media and the fact that Alzheimer's disease is a household word, some families tacitly assume that an aging relative has Alzheimer's disease without having the person examined by a medical doctor or without the knowledge that dementia has many causes and that it may be a temporary condition. Families may then begin to behave as though their relative does have the disease, initiating contact with professionals and seeking care or services for that reason. Other families may have encountered strong resistance or refusal from their relative to cooperate with a visit to a doctor. Some may have taken the person to a physician, who says that there is a likelihood that the older relative has Alzheimer's disease based on his or her age and changes in memory, behavior, or self-care. Some physicians may be operating from insufficient or incorrect information or bias, or may assume a diagnosis of probable Alzheimer's disease without obtaining a full history, completing a thorough examination, and performing appropriate tests to arrive at a correct clinical diagnosis.

Some families have been told by their physician or have heard from friends or neighbors that there is no specific test to diagnose Alzheimer's disease until autopsy. Other physicians may advise families not to "put him (or her) through all those tests" because there's no cure or treatment available. In the fiscal environment of health care in the 1990s, there may be issues in the person's health plan that have an impact on diagnosis: The primary provider may not have the knowledge, skill, time, or authorization to obtain all of the necessary and appropriate diagnostic data. On initial contact with the family, staff need to verify how the diagnosis was made and to determine whether further guidance or advocacy is needed to help the family obtain an accurate diagnosis that is based on the standards of good medical practice.

Once the care provider is assured that an accurate diagnosis has been obtained, the next step is to evaluate critically what information the family has about the disease and to clarify, update, and fill in missing information. The family needs accurate information about disease progression, available treatments, and care options to proceed with decision making. Staff often find that family members' ability to make thoughtful decisions is hampered by their lack of information about the basic pathologies of Alzheimer's disease, incorrect or insufficient information, myths, or unduly negative or catastrophic views about the disease. Many families rely on widely used, ill-defined descriptions of stages of Alzheimer's disease. It is common for families to ask, "What stage is he or she in?" When health care providers answer this question, they often disregard the extreme variability of disease progression and the impact of this language on family members' perception, expectations, and choice of care. Despite clinical experience since the 1970s that has demonstrated the positive impact of skillful communication, activities, and interactions, many families are unaware that good care practices can make an enormous difference in the level of function of their relative. Therefore, the kind and level of care their relative may benefit from also is affected.

Most families are grateful when clinicians convey a realistic hope that there are many things that can be done to improve the care and quality of life of their loved one. It is crucial for them to hear the message that although there is no medical treatment or cure for Alzheimer's disease, there are many kinds of care that can make living with the disease more tolerable, even rewarding. These types of conversations and opportunities for growth and support must take place throughout the relationship and develop through time. They also need to be appropriate to the specific family partnership and approach to care.

Many family caregivers end up at a particular care setting in a very serendipitous way. The language used to describe many care options is new and lacks clear definition. As health care institutions are in a rapid state of flux, many families no longer have access to knowledgeable clinical staff to explain the range of clinical options, admission requirements, costs, and the basis on which to make care decisions. Although there are specific information and referral services available, many families have not been linked to these services. In other cases, families have received copious amounts of information and need help in sorting through lists of resources. With the speed of health care changes, many resource lists can be incomplete or filled with omissions or inaccuracies.

Other families are highly sophisticated shoppers. They have researched, developed a short list of possible options, and cross-checked resources thoroughly. For many, the Internet has enabled them to speed through the search. Despite the rich choices, these families may not be emotionally prepared and may need help distinguishing the element of quality among their choices. Others are quite confident and present themselves at the intake assessment armed with incisive questions and a critical ear for facile answers. Staff must be sensitive to the reality of increasingly educated consumers and must be able to distinguish their care setting from other similar care settings that are competing for the family's business. Many families will make their choices based on the quality of the interaction with and impression of direct care staff with whom they first come in contact.

Exploring existing knowledge and expectations is an evolving process that must continue throughout the course of disease and care. Reviewing and reintroducing

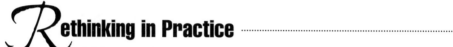

## *R*ethinking in Practice

*Talking with families about what they know about dementia and care*

*Families may have been introduced to limited or inaccurate information on Alzheimer's disease and care. Therefore, we need to spend time talking with families to explore what they know and believe and then gradually introduce a more accurate and balanced view of the disease and care. Consider the following topic areas and questions as you talk with families:*

### Diagnosis

When, where, and by whom did your relative receive a diagnosis of probable Alzheimer's disease?
What were you told about the disease?
What questions did you have that went unanswered?

### Disease Process

What do you know about the disease progression?
How did you learn about the disease course?
What are your expectations or what do you anticipate happening as the disease progresses?

### Care Approaches

What do you know about caring for someone with Alzheimer's disease?
Where did you learn about different approaches?
Which approaches have been most helpful and why?

### Care Options

What options are you aware of for care and support?
How were they introduced to you?
How did you make decisions?

### Resources

What types of resources have been most helpful to you?
Are there any specific books, videos, brochures, or other materials that have been extremely helpful to you?

knowledge and beliefs about Alzheimer's disease is an ongoing process and can lend itself to new ways of supporting families and exploring possibilities and solutions. When families are aware of the full, balanced view of Alzheimer's disease rather than only the negative aspects or limited options, they can make their own informed choices. Those individual choices or decisions then must be supported by care providers.

## WORKING WITH FAMILIES TO EXPLORE POSSIBILITIES AND FIND THEIR OWN SOLUTIONS

An abundance of literature exists on the stress and burden of caregiving but little that suggests that positive outcomes can result from the caregiving experience. Many families share stories of gratification and growth and the opportunity to find satisfaction and meaning as they grew, even in the face of challenges. When exploring the caregiving experience, we should inquire about the ways in which many families have achieved a sense of lasting pride in the newfound aspects of their relationships. In addition, we must recognize families' accomplishments resulting from becoming less judgmental and more creative, flexible, and balanced in their approach to life. Some describe growth in patience and humility, developed in the provision of steadfast daily care. Others discuss the expansion of their character and spiritual self, whereas others have described positive and deeply healing emotional experiences in relationships that were troubled.

Family caregivers often share that, after the initial shock and turmoil resulting from learning the diagnosis, they have found a way to accept the illness as an opportunity to take what is given and to fashion new kinds of relationships. Many describe a quiet but growing awareness that in living within the family crucible of Alzheimer's disease, one can dispense with old losses and grudges, put aside pettiness and bitterness, and start anew. Some caregivers reveal that at some point in this journey they reframe what is happening to them and perceive role changes as a challenge and a chance to construct a new reality. They begin to trust their own instincts and to see not just a problem but also the potential for solution. They try to avoid the temptation to focus on loss and instead look at how they can work with the qualities and remaining capacities of their relative.

In his classic book *Man's Search for Meaning*, Victor Frankl (1984) contended that every person has the potential to find meaning within his or her circumstance. Although he did not specifically discuss people with dementia, he clearly meant every person regardless of his or her abilities or disabilities. In many families, family members continue to maintain meaningful relationships with the person with dementia. For example, Elaine described the pleasure of seeing a side of her mother Ruby that she never saw before the onset of her mother's dementia (see Chapter Eight). Without the censor within her dictating her way of communication, Ruby became much more spontaneous and direct. Her daughter saw a hidden strength that was buried within her mother. In other families, a son spoke about the chance to give and receive an affectionate touch with his father; a wife heard her husband express his love and affection and gratitude for her help, something she had longed for but did not hear until she became his vital link to the world. Others perceive caring for a relative with Alzheimer's as a chance to lovingly repay a debt of gratitude or as the chance to give back to a beloved family member. One often hears a variation on the theme, "I had the chance to become better, not bitter, by choosing consciously to live in the now, not in the past." A family's perception of the disease and its impact on the person will greatly affect the meaning of providing care. Often, families are aware of the capacity of their family member with dementia to cultivate meaningful relationships, and they express frustration with health care providers who treat their family member as a nonperson.

## PROVIDING SUPPORT TO FAMILIES ALONG THE WAY

Many families value the opportunity to talk through the emotionally charged decisions that they must make as the disease progresses or just to talk about everyday experiences and struggles. It is important that we not reduce all of the needs of caregivers to those of stress and guilt. There is an enormous range and depth to the thoughts and feelings of families and the consequences of their actions and decisions. Therefore, it helps to clarify what a particular family needs from staff and the care setting. Support and guidance may be facilitated by the setting but may actually be provided in a variety of innovative ways. Families may have a natural bond with someone on staff because of their unique background, chemistry, or other such factors. It is important for staff to put the needs of the family first and to determine who can best meet those needs. Staff members may facilitate resolution for a family that is "stuck" by holding an informal meeting with another caregiver who has worked through a similar dilemma. On other occasions, the need may be met best by engaging the family to provide some volunteer hours on a field trip, where a caregiver may see role-modeling of communication techniques in action, although role modeling was not the stated (but was the intended) purpose.

Some families have support needs that challenge staff to provide or facilitate support in unique and nontraditional ways. Many family caregivers are referred to support groups but never consider the option because they feel it is out of character. They may not be comfortable sharing their emotions in public or may become overwhelmed by the prospect of incontinence or changes in hygiene. Some caregivers say that their own burden is so great that they cannot also bear the weight of another's burden. Others find there is too much negativity or griping in these groups. Other families may feel that family business is private and should not be aired in public or that it would dishonor the person to speak ill of him or her in front of strangers.

It may help to ask families directly what kind of support they think would best fit their needs. They may be able to ask for the kind of help that is needed on a situational basis, such as for someone to visit residential facilities with them or how to respond to other family members who may be critical of decisions made. Families may need permission to express their feelings to others who will not be shocked by what they may say. Some may seek affirmation that their care is skillful, although problems may persist. Others may appreciate a chance to talk about the joys in their life or share in their satisfaction at obtaining their driver's license at age 67. Other families may appreciate hearing that humor (i.e., laughing with, not at, their relative) is a common and legitimate way to ease daily frustrations. Some families may feel helpless in the face of the dementing illness and may welcome the chance to provide testimony before a legislative committee on a bill that would fund additional research programs. Others may welcome the opportunity to share a social event with their spouse and other couples who are dealing with dementia, to maintain a feeling of normalcy. Whatever the case, the type, amount, and means of support varies from family to family and individual to individual.

## BALANCING PERSON-CENTERED CARE WITHIN THE CONTEXT OF A FAMILY-CENTERED APPROACH

There are times when the needs or wishes of a family may conflict with the needs and wishes of the person with dementia. In these situations clinicians often get caught in the middle because of the difficulty in balancing the conflicting needs and wishes. Sometimes these situations may seem fairly arbitrary, but often it is possible to reach a compromise that is satisfactory to those involved. For example, Bill's wife

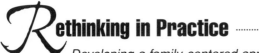

# *R*ethinking in Practice

*Developing a family-centered approach to care*

> *To develop an approach that is appropriate for a particular family, it is important to understand what that family believes and how they function. Think about a specific family and try to gain an understanding of how their system functions. Consider the following questions as you learn more about the system:*

Who are the members of the family system?
How does the system function?
How do they handle illness?
How do they cope with change?
How are they involved in care?
What are their strengths and needs?
What are their expectations?
What do they know about Alzheimer's disease and care?
How familiar are they with their options?
What type of support do they want and/or need?
How familiar are they with different possibilities?
Which type of partnership are they comfortable with?

> *It may be helpful to spend some time developing a specific plan for the family on how to work with and support them in providing person-centered care.*

Sarah was distressed because he often spilled food and could not maintain his life-long need for tidiness. Her solution was to insist that he wear a bib. He did not like the bib and resisted using it. In a staff discussion about the situation options were explored, and the staff tried an alternative that proved satisfactory to both Bill and Sarah: When getting ready for a meal, a staff member offered plastic aprons to Bill and other individuals and put one on herself. Bill no longer felt that he was "being treated like a baby," and his wife was not distressed by his appearance after meals.

Although balancing conflicting needs is not always so simply resolved, the principles of resolution are essentially the same and begin by defining the problem. Sarah was distressed by his appearance, but he did not seem aware of or distressed by his drips and spills. Bill was distressed by the bib. This raises questions about who really has the problem. Some staff felt that the problem was Sarah's concerns about Bill's lack of tidiness. Others felt that the problem was his expressed feelings about wearing a bib. Still other staff members believed that the problem was how to deal with Sarah's anger with staff when Bill refused to wear the bib. If in such an everyday matter it is not easy to clearly define the problem, then we can appreciate the difficulty of defining the problem in more complex situations.

Sometimes it is necessary to move to "the next step," considering all of the facts and looking at the situation from a variety of perspectives before staff can clearly articulate the problem. In considering two clearly expressed but differing positions, such as the feelings of Bill and his wife, it is important not to get caught in an either–or thought process. In exploring the possible motives and values for each position, staff learned that this was not primarily an issue of control for Sarah or of autonomy for Bill but rather an issue of personal dignity for both Bill and his wife. Sarah knew that Bill would have been embarrassed had he been aware of the stains on his shirt after lunch. She also was concerned about how this change in his personal habits would affect relationships with friends and relatives. In her efforts to help him maintain his characteristic tidiness, she lost perspective about how wearing a bib made him feel. It was only after exploring the situation from differing perspectives that the actual problem was clearly defined, and this helped Bill to maintain his dignity during and after meals. In more complex situations, the facts and perspectives may go beyond the feelings and concerns of the person, the family, and the staff. Legal, professional, and care-setting responsibilities may need to be considered to gain as full an understanding of a situation as possible.

As options and alternatives to resolve a situation are considered, it is important to weigh the likely outcome of each possible alternative solution because many actions have unintended or unanticipated consequences. It may even be helpful to list those parties involved to help determine how each party will be affected by the different alternatives being considered. The primary goal for staff is to meet the needs of the person with dementia. Because that person does not exist in a vacuum, staff must make the effort to meet those needs in a way that recognizes the context of the person's life and supports the relationships involved.

Given the social fabric of each person's life, the necessity of helping the person maintain the family connections that are part of his or her social identity becomes readily apparent. Maintaining these connections often requires helping family members think in somewhat different ways about these relationships. Some adult children will talk about role changes, saying, "I'm the mother now; sometimes she even calls me 'Mother'." Although a person with dementia may call a child by another person's name, he or she is still the parent and gets pleasure from having that relationship acknowledged and even celebrated.

Maintaining these connections also may require that staff think in different ways about the importance of these relationships. Sometimes staff members who are especially close to a person with dementia will say, "We are her family now." This negates family relationships that are still important, even if these relationships are strained, severed, or only partially remembered. Even in very difficult family relationships, there is usually some part of the relationship that is important to the person and that needs to be acknowledged to help the person maintain his or her social identity. As clinicians we need to be alert to the significance of family relationships for the person with dementia and find ways to work with family members to nourish and support the meaning of that relationship. Many, if not most, families need the help of a variety of care providers to support and supplement, not supplant, the family's efforts. The social context of care for the person with dementia cannot be limited to the milieu of the care setting. It also must include the family relationships that have been and continue to be a significant part of the person's life.

## REFERENCES

Bowen, M. (1971). The use of family theory in clinical practice. In J. Haley (Ed.), *Changing families* (pp. 159–191). New York: Grune & Stratton.

Foley, V. (1974). *An introduction to family therapy.* New York: Grune & Stratton.

Frank, L.R. (Ed.). (1995). *Influencing minds: A reader in quotations* (p. 216). Portland, OR: Feral House (Kissinger quotation originally appeared in his 1982 book *Years of Upheaval*).

Frankl, V. (1984). *Man's search for meaning.* New York: Simon & Schuster.

McDaniel, S.H., Hepworth, J., & Doherty, W.J. (1992). *Medical family therapy: A biopsychosocial approach to families with health problems.* New York: Basic Books.

Orange, J. (1991). Perspectives of family members regarding communication changes. In R. Lubinski (Ed.), *Dementia and communication* (pp. 168–186). Philadelphia: B.C. Decker.

Rolland, J.S. (1994). *Families, illness & disability: An integrative treatment model.* New York: Basic Books.

# $\mathcal{R}$einvesting in Alzheimer's Care

*Unless someone like you cares a whole awful lot,*
*Nothing is going to get better.*
*It's not.*

*Dr. Seuss,* The Lorax

During the 1990s, interest in ways to improve care for people with dementia has grown, and many clinicians, researchers, and people with dementia and their family members have shared a variety of information about the disease, the experience of the disease, and care provision. As understanding of some of the needs of people with dementia and their families has increased, programs have been developed in response to those needs. Although there are a number of special care units and programs for people with dementia, it is not altogether clear what is "special" about the care or programs or how the quality of life for the person with dementia has been improved. Perhaps one of the reasons that it has been difficult to explain clearly what is special about these programs is what Deming (1982) described as a lack of a constancy of purpose—the lack of a clear definition of and focus on what we are trying to accomplish. With all of the information being generated about providing care for people with dementia, the pieces of information have yet to be organized into a coherent whole or a single body of knowledge incorporating the many diverse parts. Given the state of knowledge, it is easy to get lost in the trees and lose sight of the forest.

Although dementia is a degenerative disease that is debilitating in many ways, people with dementia "normalize" the disease or incorporate it into their lives, rather than use it to define themselves. This incorporation supports the assertion that despite the problems a person experiences because of changes caused by the disease, he or she can still "be in a state of at least relative well-being" and that maintenance of the individual's personhood is dependent on the quality of interpersonal interactions experienced (Kitwood & Bredin, 1992, p. 270). It also provides a clear framework and direction for us as clinicians. Our purpose is to help the person with dementia maintain his or her sense of well-being by recognizing and focusing on the person rather than identifying and focusing on the symptoms of the disease.

If we accept the premise that the personhood of an individual with dementia can be enhanced or compromised by the quality and character of interpersonal interactions, then we must focus attention and energy on the person's social environment. Like many clinicians, Lyman (1989) has long contended that it is the social context of care rather than the biological losses of a person that most affect how the disease is experienced. Because we are social beings, almost everything we do occurs in the context of a social system, whether at home or in a group care setting. Rethinking the way that care for people with dementia is provided requires thought about the system of care and consideration of the parts of the system that support or hinder a commitment to good-quality care.

## UNDERSTANDING SYSTEMS AS THE CONTEXT OF CARE FOR PEOPLE WITH DEMENTIA

Serious consideration of the social context of care means that attention must be paid to the whole system of care, not just small pieces of the system. Many system theorists believe that it is not possible to understand a system by looking only at its parts. The whole is greater than the sum of the parts because of the synergy created when all parts of a system or environment of care work together to support the same goals. Thus, to understand a system, we must have an appreciation of the whole system, its position in larger systems, and the relationships within the system (Capra, 1996). Systems theory also can be used as a means of understanding the change we experience, individually and collectively. It is especially important to recognize that any change in a system, regardless of how large or small, will result in a change in other parts of the system.

Scientists, from physicists to biologists to social scientists, contend that all systems are dynamic and in a continuous state of change or evolution. These are the incremental changes that we are accustomed to and that are characterized by words such as "grow," "develop," "evolve," "learn," and "adapt" (Kelly, 1994). Sometimes in social systems there is change of such magnitude that words such as "revolutionary" or "reformation" are used to describe it. Traditionally, periods of great change, such as the Industrial Revolution, also were periods of great strife with long periods of adaptation. In the late 20th century, large-magnitude changes occur with such frequency that efforts are made to structure systems to incorporate change and to minimize distress and disruption and hasten adaptation. The saying that "there are two things certain in this life, death and taxes" should be amended to there are three things certain in this life—death, taxes, and change.

Throughout the 1990s major changes have occurred in virtually every aspect of health care. It is not yet clear what the constellation of health and social services will look like or how the parts will fit together. The very foundations are being rearranged. The emerging system cannot be understood by relying on traditional definitions and ways of doing things. This is, as we sense it, not a tinkering around the edges but a revolutionary change. Almost everyone in the field of health and social services has seen the traditional ways of thinking about people, disease, and care being questioned. How, where, and by whom care is provided has and will continue to change fundamentally.

In times of great change, there is both great uncertainty and great opportunity. When staff receive little information and do not know how to interpret what these changes might mean for their program and themselves, feelings of powerlessness often crop up. When leaders help translate trends into understandable terms, a common language and framework are provided for considering events in factual ways that minimize anxiety and maximize problem-solving responses. By putting health care changes in a historical perspective, it is possible to see reasons for change, to understand the factors that impinge on the present situation, and to identify the forces that affect us and may affect us. Managed well, this continuous open interpretation and discussion of factors that influence the larger systems of which we are a part can be a source for ongoing renewal, a vital element for the reinvigoration of staff and the organization. This continuous flow of information provides an evolving frame of reference that puts providing care for people with dementia in a larger context.

## REVITALIZING SYSTEMS OF CARE

Revitalization can be thought of as the infusion of life, energy, attentiveness, connection, and sustained focus on the provision of care. This concept seems both somewhat elusive to define and easily recognizable. Each of us has witnessed the contrast among staff members as they go about their work: Some seem to be on automatic pilot, going through the motions of providing care, appearing to have little invest-

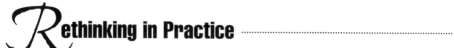

## *R*ethinking in Practice

*Understanding the impact of the changing system of care*

*It is important to understand the impact of the whole system and changes in the system on the context of care. We must understand the interconnections of all of the components to identify ways the system is or is not supportive of the person with dementia. With a clear understanding of the system as a whole, we can determine ways to modify the context of care to be more supportive of the person with dementia.*

What changes in the health care system as a whole have had the most direct impact on a care setting you know?
How have these changes affected you personally?
What changes have affected the way that care is provided?
Have these changes had a positive or negative impact on older people with dementia?
Is the quality of life of older people with dementia all that it could be? Is more change needed to support a sense of well-being for them?

ment. Watching them work, one observes people who do not seem to put much effort into or get much out of their job. In interactions with individuals or within groups, some staff could just as easily be interacting with inanimate objects. Their body language seems robotic and mechanical.

Other staff seem to be fully present. All of their senses seem fully engaged (e.g., good eye contact, listen for subtle sounds, attentive and attuned to the body language of the person with dementia). They seem to be receptive to the person and responsive to the person's needs. There seems to be an easy give-and-take, an exchange, a familiarity, and a warmth. There often is mutual greeting and touching and other small gestures of acceptance or shared affection. The interactions seem to be about much more than just the specific tasks, reflecting pleasure in sharing.

The first description of staff illustrates an absence of vitality; the second illuminates the presence of a kind of energy that changes the care experience for the person providing care, the person receiving care, and those who witness the interactions. There seem to be some important and fundamental differences in the ways that these staff, who have such contrasting styles, approach relationships. All too often one hears staff who connect with others and display pride and pleasure in their work described as "special people." Some people may be naturally more empathic, caring, outgoing, or expressive than others; however, it is unfair to other staff and people with dementia if these characteristics are simply regarded as innate, and no effort is made to help others reach the same level of performance.

In systems theory emphasis is placed on determining what parts in the system either help or hinder staff in attaining peak performance rather than on blaming the individual staff member or the task. The first example of staff members raises a number of questions for even the most casual observer: How does such a person relate to others outside work? Does this person even see people with dementia or think his or her work performance does not matter because they can't remember? What does the person think the work of providing care is about—being on time and completing all of the assigned tasks? How was this person oriented to the work of caregiving? Was the importance of validating relationships emphasized? What evaluation standards have been established for this person? What gratification is there for either the provider of care or the recipient of care? This example shows that in this setting care is used as a noun and not as a verb. When the lack of caring (verb) is as evident as in the first example, we can conclude only that caring (verb) is not a value or a commitment of the leadership in this setting.

In settings like that in the first vignette, it is common to hear litanies of the difficulties of working with people with dementia. The work is described as incredibly stressful, resulting in burnout that accounts for the frequent staff turnover in the organization. When one listens closely to the staff's complaints, however, it is clear that many of the problems that staff are experiencing are problems in the system that are unrelated to the person with dementia (e.g., short staffing due to vacant positions, staff with little knowledge about dementia). Although the organization's leadership may not consciously encourage blaming the difficulties staff are experiencing on the person with dementia, this is often the result if the issues are not acknowledged and addressed as organizational problems.

There often are complaints from leadership about the poor quality of the work pool and the difficulty of finding good workers, who are kind and do not mind doing all of the difficult things that need to be done. These "good" and "kind" workers are perceived as having emerged into the world with those qualities. They are seen as exceptional or special people who somehow have found ways to handle even the most difficult person with dementia. They often are described as committed and dedicated. Although these positive qualities may appear innate, it is likely that their sensitivity was learned in other work settings or through their personal life and relationships. Commitment is a personal attribute that certainly cannot be mandated for others; however, leadership in any organization can and must establish clear expectations about how care is to be provided by all staff, not just those "special," "good," or "kind" workers. These expectations must be followed with the implementation of a plan to develop, guide, and mentor all staff to help each person reach his or her potential. In this way, the whole system of care can be revitalized, and staff can exhibit the qualities of vitality, enthusiasm, and affection that foster real connections with people with dementia.

## EXPLORING ORGANIZATIONAL COMMITMENT

Deming was one of the leading proponents of having respect for the abilities and capacity of staff to make positive contributions to the goals of an organization. Although he was ardently opposed to fear-producing management tactics, he was equally ardent about making clear expectations about appropriate actions and an "awareness of consequences of intolerable actions" (Deming, 1982). He contended that this approach is not fear-producing in staff but provides an environment that supports personal growth and creativity.

Given the impact of interpersonal interactions on the well-being of the person with dementia, expectations about the quality of interpersonal skills and interactions should be made clear to every staff member who has contact with an older person with dementia. Training in ways to achieve the goal of having every interpersonal interaction validate the person with dementia should be provided. The training must be incorporated into the staff's daily practices, and it must be reinforced through role-modeling by formal and informal leaders. To further ensure that the importance of interpersonal interaction is recognized as a critical job skill, specific types of desired communication skills should be included in the evaluation standards for each staff member.

If the leadership, both formal and informal, is committed to living a philosophy of care (see Chapter Two) that is based on validating and respecting the person with dementia, everyone in the organization will more closely resemble the staff described in the second example on page 158. If continuously improving the way that care is provided is a clear expectation of the organization's leadership, both leadership and staff will make the effort to find ways to accomplish this. If leadership is committed to focusing effort on attaining outcomes, such as having the person with dementia express affection and have fun, then staff would be expected to interact warmly and respectfully with people with dementia, enjoy these interactions, and express pride in what they are doing. Focusing the attention and efforts of everyone in the system on achieving outcomes that are based on the organization's philosophy of care will benefit not only the person with dementia but also the entire organization.

Having and articulating clear expectations to help every staff member develop necessary interpersonal and care skills is important to the organization and to the person with dementia. If the organization depends solely on "good" staff, then when they leave the organization the culture of caring goes with them. Staff who are nurtured and encouraged to grow personally and professionally are more likely to be more creative about improving ways to provide care. Acknowledging excellence and sharing positive feedback from families and visitors publicly, such as in staff meetings and in private conversations with staff, emphasize the importance of caring to the organization. The synergy that results from staff who are growing in skill and ability to connect with people with dementia produces an energy and vibrancy that affects everyone in an organization.

## EVALUATING PERSONAL COMMITMENT

Although care is provided within the context of a system, it is accomplished through the interactions of individuals. Organizational leaders can establish expectations

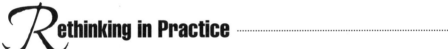

## *R*ethinking in Practice

*Assessing organizational commitment*

*If an organization's purpose is to help the person with dementia sustain a state of well-being by recognizing and focusing on the person rather than identifying and focusing on the symptoms of this disease, then a number of organizational paradigms may need to change. Although real and sustained change requires true commitment from leadership, every person in the organization needs to be involved in the process of planning and implementing the change.*

*Using personal and collective experience as data, "the way we've always done it" must be questioned and challenged. Ask yourself and others the following questions:*

Why is care, such as the way meals are served or personal care, being provided the way it is now?

How do people with dementia respond to current caregiving methods?

*Think of some instances in which people responded positively or exhibited signs of well-being. Building on these positive experiences, consider some possible solutions to old problems.*

What are some ways to support the positive efforts of staff and reduce or eliminate the situations that drain staff energy?

What suggestions do people with dementia and/or their family members have to make care provision more supportive of the person with dementia?

When visiting dementia programs, what ideas or ways of doing things have you seen that can be adapted to your setting?

about the nature of interactions, and commitment can be encouraged, but commitment is a personal decision. It is an internal process based on a person's value system and beliefs about people with dementia. The intrinsic motivation for this commitment comes from the importance of the work itself and enriching connections. Commitment does not mean simply to do a good job or to be a good employee but to relate to each person with dementia and to try to understand the person's point of view and experience.

We must begin by honestly evaluating the way that we think about people with dementia. Each person has different caregiving and life experiences with people with dementia. These experiences and our beliefs color our perception of the person with dementia. To accept and be committed to the belief that we can help mitigate the impact of the disease and help the person maintain a state of well-being means different sorts of journeys for each of us. For some it is a validation of a belief held but that perhaps cannot be clearly articulated. Others may not have thought about people with dementia in this way before and may need to begin to change a number of beliefs about them, from loss to ability, from care to contribution, and from burden to benefit. Still others may have been advocates of this belief for some time but have gotten into a rut and need an infusion of energy. Other people may be at critical points between those described. Because each of us starts in different places, the journey to make personal changes is different for each of us. The journey is rewarding when we fully recognize how knowing people with dementia has enriched our lives and acknowledge the personal growth that results from connected relationships. A Chinese proverb says, "A journey of a thousand miles begins with a single step."

This process of changing perspective comes easier to some people than to others. Although the capacity for self-awareness and self-reflection is developed individually, many people may be helped in the process by sharing the journey with others. It often is helpful to identify others with similar beliefs, to share thoughts, feelings, and experiences and receive honest and supportive feedback. This exchange may provide the perspective that is necessary to determine what shifts in our thinking are needed and the ways that these shifts might be accomplished. Some caregivers must unlearn ways that were taught and question negative views and stereotypes. Many of these reactions may be so subtle and powerful that we are not even aware of how they have influenced our thinking and behavior.

As discussed in Chapter One, the language used may frame the people who have dementia and those who care for them in very negative terms. Negative language may affect our approach to care in ways that cause us to feel defeated before we begin to provide it. Negative perceptions may color the way that we view the people we care for, ourselves, and the work that we do. If we appraise what we do honestly and find that barriers to connecting with the person with dementia exist, then we can begin to identify ways to overcome them.

As we begin to be more sensitive to the behaviors that indicate well-being in the person with dementia, we likely will begin to make changes in our practice, creating a cycle of success for both the person with dementia and ourselves. Some people may find this increase in personal satisfaction rewarding enough to sustain a personal commitment, regardless of the surrounding culture or system. Others may want to share this experience more generally or may want and need feedback from others to guide changes in their practice. For these people it is critical to understand the system and to assess accurately what is necessary to make changes within a system. A mentor outside the organization may be able to guide growth and provide supportive and realistic feedback about change in a system.

Because organizations are in some ways like an Alexander Calder mobile (when one part changes all of the parts are affected by the change), Deming (1982) contended that it is possible to initiate change in a system from multiple positions within an organization. This does not mean that all parts change in the same way or that changes in one part mirror the change in other parts. It is also important to recognize that in an organization, movement is not necessarily an indicator of real change.

Position and understanding of the system can determine the speed with which change occurs and the effort involved in bringing about a desired change. It may be that there are enough people in an organization who want to provide care in this more connected way, to form the necessary "critical mass" to effect a real organizational transformation. It may be that there are not adequate numbers of people who want to bring about real change, or it may be such an uphill struggle that the effort needed is beyond one person's resources. Rather than try to move an immovable object, a person may decide that a satisfying personal experience is sustaining enough. Alternatively, a person may choose the option of modeling the desired

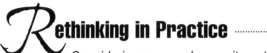

# ethinking in Practice

### Considering personal commitment

*It is critical that the staff and leadership of health care programs identify and nurture, in themselves and others, the qualities that convey a sense of connection, caring, respect, and validation to older adults with dementia. Reflect on what gives you the strength and purpose to bring your highest level of effort to working with people with dementia each day. Describe and compare some of those sources of energy with your colleagues and co-workers.*

What are some of the things outside of yourself that encourage you to put forth your best effort?

Can you describe a time when you felt vulnerable and had to rely on someone else to assist you? What was that experience like? How did the different approaches of others affect you?

When we give 100% to our interactions with people with dementia, what effect does it have on them? When we give less than 100%?

What situations in your work environment create energy and enthusiasm? What situations in your work environment drain your energy? What brings you real joy?

What are some ways to maximize the situations that give you energy or to change the situations that sap your energy? If the energy-draining situations are not within your power to change, then in what ways could you diminish the negative impact?

change, which can be an effective, if slow, mechanism to promote change; or he or she may choose to find an organization that is more compatible with his or her beliefs and practices. Personal and professional situations guide these choices, but the connection with people with dementia provides personal satisfaction regardless of the practice setting.

Many people who are caring for people with dementia resist describing their role as a burden because they find it to be so meaningful and fulfilling. Not only are interpersonal relationships critical to sustaining a sense of personhood and well-being for the person with dementia but these relationships also sustain and enhance the personhood and well-being of the people who care for them. This leads some caregivers to describe caring for a person with dementia as a sometimes challenging but life-enriching and transforming experience.

## INCREASING SOCIETAL COMMITMENT

The Alzheimer's Association and many advocates, families, and professionals have worked tirelessly to make U.S. society, as a whole, aware of the needs of people with Alzheimer's disease and their families. In a relatively short time period, this massive effort has been enormously successful. This effort brought the needs of people with dementia to the attention of not only the public but also to organizations, which responded by creating programs to address a wide variety of these needs. Public policy efforts brought an infusion of money for research. The achievements to develop public awareness and support for programs for people with dementia since the 1970s are truly remarkable.

Bringing the scope of the problems faced by people with dementia and their families to the public's attention and gaining support for public policy changes required stressing the negative aspects of the disease. Detailing all of the problems caused by the disease and stressing negativity were necessary to educate legislators about the needs as advocates and researchers competed for scarce resources. Although these efforts certainly helped bring about needed changes, a very negative image of dementia has been created. We need to find ways to change the public perception from this solely negative image to a more balanced understanding of the experience of the disease for both people with dementia and their families.

To advance public awareness to a real societal commitment for supporting the person with dementia requires a willingness to work toward change as private citizens, taxpayers, and members of professional organizations. There is much that we can do that can have a positive impact on people with dementia. We can write letters to the editors of newspapers if coverage of dementia is too negative, correct myths and misstatements of facts among friends and neighbors discussing Alzheimer's disease, offer to write an article for a local newsletter, or suggest speakers for community organizations of which we are members. If we consider what has been accomplished to this point, then taking these achievements to the next level is a realistic goal, especially if we follow the advice of the Chinese proverb, "To move a mountain, begin with carrying a single stone."

## UNDERSTANDING WHY COMMITMENT MATTERS

Real and universal change is needed in providing care for older adults with dementia. The many positive changes in how and where care is provided have been more incremental than revolutionary—in some settings and not others, with some but not all staff members. More important, as our understanding of the experience of dementia has grown, although it is yet incomplete, it is adequate to provide a framework for practice. We can learn from the experience of numerous clinicians, both published and unpublished. The basic message is the same: Recognize and connect with the person with dementia rather than focus on the symptoms of the disease.

There is an enormous need for change in almost all areas of care for older people with dementia. The variety of care settings does not meet current needs, nor will it be sufficient to meet population projections in subsequent generations. Population studies show that older adults are the fastest-growing segment of the U.S. population. Research also shows that Alzheimer's disease affects nearly 50% of people age 85 and older (Evans et al., 1989). With the incidence of dementia virtually doubling in each successive generation, there is an urgent need to expand the knowledge of the disease and ways of mitigating its impact on people with the illness and their families. There is also a compelling need to translate knowledge into action in all settings and increase the availability of programs and services for this large and diverse population.

The earlier that we can acknowledge and accept the challenge of change, the more likely we are to succeed in implementing the programs that are needed. The values that guide and shape the necessary array of programs and services are determined by the people who are the most committed and become the strongest advocates. Those of us who truly and passionately believe that caring for and connecting

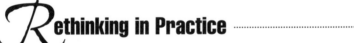

# *R*ethinking in Practice

*Shifting from public awareness to public commitment*

*The following questions may help you to reflect on the shifts in focus needed in our efforts to create a real societal commitment to care for people with dementia.*

How do you think the public perceives people with Alzheimer's disease? How does that perception compare with staff experience in working with people with dementia?

Why do those differences in perception exist? What can be done to make perceptions of the disease more accurate?

How does the public view your job? What do you think your job is?

How much has the knowledge about Alzheimer's disease changed since you began working with people with dementia? Are your acquaintances and friends outside work aware of these advances? Have regulatory policies changed rules based on this knowledge?

Has the way that care is provided for people with dementia changed since you began working in this field? What changes are needed in your care setting in order to take caregiving to the next level and be truly supportive of people with dementia?

with people with dementia is critical in any setting or service must be actively engaged in the effort to influence the future of dementia care. As has been said, "The best way to predict the future is to create it" (author unknown).

## REFERENCES

Capra, F. (1996). *The web of life.* New York: Anchor Books.

Deming, W.E. (1982). *Out of crisis.* Cambridge: Massachusetts Institute of Technology, Center for Advanced Engineering Study.

Evans, D., Funkenstein, H.H., Albert, M.S., Scherr, P.K., Cook, N.R., Chonwn, M.J., Herbert, L.E., Hennekens, C.H., & Taylor, J.D. (1989). Prevalence of Alzheimer's disease in a community population higher than previously reported. *Journal of the American Medical Association, 262,* 2251–2256.

Geisel, T. (Dr. Seuss). (1971). *The lorax.* New York: Random House.

Kelly, K. (1994). *Out of control.* Reading, MA: Perseus Books.

Kitwood, T., & Bredin, K. (1992). Towards a theory of dementia care: Personhood and well being. *Aging and Society, 12,* 269–287.

Lyman, K.A. (1989). Bringing the social back in: A critique of the biomedicalization of dementia. *Gerontologist, 29,* 597–605.

# ℛ ecommended Readings

Aguilera, D.C., & Messick, J.M. (1986). *Crisis intervention: Theory and methodology.* St. Louis: Mosby.

Bell, V., & Troxel, D. (1997). *The best friends approach to Alzheimer's care.* Baltimore: Health Professions Press.

Binstock, R.H., Post, S., & Whitehouse, P.J. (1992). *Dementia and aging: Ethics, values and policy choices.* Baltimore: The Johns Hopkins University Press.

Boss, P. (1999). *Ambiguous loss: Learning to live with unresolved grief.* Cambridge, MA: Harvard University Press.

Brandon, D. (1990). *Zen in the art of helping.* New York: Arkana.

Capra, F. (1991). *The tao of physics.* Boston: Shambhala.

Carlson, R., & Shield, B. (Eds.). (1995). *Handbook for the soul.* Boston: Little, Brown.

Carse, J.P. (1994). *Breakfast at the victory: The mysticism of ordinary experience.* New York: HarperCollins.

Chopra, D. (1992). *Unconditional life.* New York: Bantam Books.

Cousineau, P. (Ed.). (1994). *Soul: An archaeology.* New York: HarperCollins.

Davidson, A. (1997). *Alzheimer's, a love story: One year in my husband's journey.* Secaucus, NJ: Carol Publishing.

Dawson, P., Wells, D.L., & Kline, K. (1993). *Enhancing the abilities of persons with Alzheimer's and related dementias.* New York: Springer.

Dossey, L. (1993). *Healing words: The power of prayer and the practice of medicine.* New York: HarperCollins.

Farran, C.J., Herth, K.A., & Popovich, J.M. (1995). *Hope and hopelessness: Critical clinical constructs.* Beverly Hills, CA: Sage Publications.

Frankl, V.E. (1959). *Man's search for meaning.* New York: Washington Square Press.

Frankl, V.E. (1986). *The doctor and the soul.* New York: Vintage Books.

Goldsmith, M. (1996). *Hearing the voices of people with dementia.* London: Jessica Kingsley Publishers.

Gunaratana, V.H. (1994). *Mindfulness in plain English.* Boston: Wisdom Publications.

Hall, E.T. (1989). *The dance of life: The other dimension of time.* New York: Anchor Books.

Hayward, J. (1995). *Sacred world.* New York: Bantam Books.

Heidegger, M. (1971). *Poetry, language, thought* (A. Hofstadter, Trans.). New York: Harper & Row.

**167**

Kabat-Zinn, J. (1994). *Wherever you go, there you are: Mindfulness meditation in everyday life.* New York: Hyperion.

Kellert, S.H. (1993). *In the wake of chaos.* Chicago: University of Chicago Press.

Kushner, L. (1996). *Invisible lines of connection: Sacred stories of the ordinary.* Woodstock, VT: Jewish Lights Publishing.

Lubkin, I.M. (1986). *Chronic illness: Impact and interventions.* Boston: Jones & Bartlett.

Lustbader, W., & Hooyman, N.R. (1994). *Taking care of aging family members: A practical guide.* New York: The Free Press.

Mayeroff, M. (1971). *On caring.* New York: Harper Perennial.

McGoldrick, M., Pearce, J.K., & Giordano, J. (Eds.). (1982). *Ethnicity & family therapy.* New York: The Guilford Press.

Mcneill, D., & Freiberger, P. (1993). *Fuzzy logic.* New York: Simon & Schuster.

Ortony, A. (Ed.) (1993). *Metaphor and thought.* New York: Cambridge University Press.

Pipher, M. (1999). *Another country: Navigating the emotional terrain of our elders.* New York: Riverhead Books.

Post, S. (1995). *The moral challenges of Alzheimer's disease.* Baltimore: The Johns Hopkins University Press.

Rader, J. (1995). *Individualized dementia care: Creative, compassionate approaches.* New York: Springer.

Rosenberg, C.E. (1987). *The care of strangers: The rise of America's hospital system.* New York: Basic Books.

Saul, J.R. (1992). *Voltaire's bastards: The dictatorship of reason in the West.* New York: Vintage Books.

Starr, P. (1982). *The social transformation of American medicine: The rise of a sovereign profession and the making of a vast industry.* New York: Basic Books.

Wilber, K. (Ed.) (1985). *Quantum questions: Mystical writings of the world's greatest physicists.* Boston: Shambhala.

Wong, P.T., & Fry, P.S. (1998). *The human quest for meaning: A handbook of psychological research and clinical applications.* Mahwah, NJ: Lawrence Erlbaum Associates.

Yeo, G., & Gallagher-Thompson, D. (Eds.). (1996). *Ethnicity and the dementias.* Washington, DC: Taylor & Francis.

Zohar, D. (1997). *Re-wiring the corporate brain: Using the new science to re-think how we structure and lead organizations.* San Francisco: Berrett-Koehler Publishers.

Zohar, D., & Marshall, I. (1994). *The quantum society.* New York: William Morrow & Company.

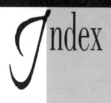
# Index

*Page references followed by f or t indicate figures or tables, respectively.*